Survival Handbook in Pediatric Surgical Oncology

Lucas Krauel
Editor

Survival Handbook in Pediatric Surgical Oncology

Springer

Editor
Lucas Krauel
Pediatric Surgical Oncology
Pediatric Surgery Department
Pediatric Cancer Center Barcelona (PCCB)
SJD Barcelona Children's Hospital
Universitat de Barcelona
Barcelona, Spain

ISBN 978-3-031-65889-1 ISBN 978-3-031-65890-7 (eBook)
https://doi.org/10.1007/978-3-031-65890-7

This Springer imprint is published by the registered company Springer Nature Switzerland AG
The registered company address is: Gewerbestrasse 11, 6330 Cham, Switzerland

Foreword

The *Survival Handbook in Pediatric Surgical Oncology* fulfills a great need for the surgeon to have a ready reference that is comprehensive, algorithm-oriented, and yet brief enough to carry to the operating room for quick reference. There is a chapter on the relevance and importance of the tumor board, and another that provides a comprehensive discussion of vascular access techniques. The approach to tumor biopsies is discussed in detail including anatomical orientation, the need for adequate tissue sampling, and the requirement to not jeopardize subsequent resection. All major tumor systems that occur in childhood and adolescence are discussed in detail and the following are included: neuroblastoma, Wilms tumor, liver tumors, gonadal tumors, sarcomas, bone tumors, thyroid tumors, and lymphoma. There is also a nice chapter on the management of enlarged lymph nodes and another that describes rare tumor of childhood including melanoma and pancreatic tumors. Further, there are additional chapters on the management of metastases, pediatric surgical emergencies, and palliative care. The timing of surgery after neoadjuvant chemotherapy is elucidated including the effect of this treatment on resectability and surgical complications. Management standards based on the results of cooperative group protocols from both the United States and Europe are emphasized. Guiding principles are supplemented by very good descriptions of surgical technique, including types of incisions and exposures. I believe this handbook will be very useful for all pediatric surgeons involved in the care of children with cancer. In addition, trainees in pediatric surgery and pediatric surgical advanced practitioners will also benefit from the abbreviated but complete descriptions of tumor management. Finally, pediatric medical oncologists may profit from the insight into surgical management of their young patients included in this text.

Joseph H. Burchenal Chair
in Pediatrics, Memorial Sloan
Kettering Cancer Center (MSKCC)
New York, NY, USA

Michael P. LaQuaglia

Contents

Pediatric Cancer and Its Singularity

1

Jaume Mora and Guillermo Chantada

1.1 Introduction

Pediatrics is the branch of medicine that deals with the medical care of infants, children, and adolescents, and the fundamental characteristic of these three stages in life is growth. Cancer is defined concisely as the territorial expansion of a mutant clone. We define pediatric cancers as those that develop during and as the consequence of the complex process of development, while body growth is active [1].

1.2 Epidemiology

An estimated 430,000 new cases of childhood cancer are expected globally each year. The age-standardized reported incidence rates are 141 per million person-years (children: 0–14 years) and 185 per million person-years (adolescents: 15–19 years). Incidence rates for children aged 0–14 years range from 59.5 per million person-years in sub-Saharan Africa to 175.1 in southern Europe (155.8 for Spain). Age-standardized incidence rate for leukemia is 49.1 per million person-years followed by CNS tumors 30.4 per million person-years [2].

Childhood cancer is substantially underdiagnosed, especially in South Asia and sub-Saharan Africa. Taking current projections of population growth into account, the estimate is that there will be 13.7 million new cases of childhood cancer worldwide from 2020 to 2050, of which around 3.4 million will be in low-income countries (LIC) and about 6.9 million in lower-middle-income countries (LMIC). In 2020–2050, the projected number of new cases of childhood cancer in upper middle-income countries will be 2.5 million, with a further 939,000 in high-income countries (HIC). Given the estimated incidence of children (0–14 years) with cancer of 430,000 worldwide (10,000 in the USA and 15,000 in Europe) in 2020, 232,000 will be diagnosed, and 181,000 will remain undiagnosed [3].

Demographic trends show that the annual incidence of childhood cancer is projected to diverge according to country income group, with HIC and upper-middle-income countries showing a decline in cases, whereas cases will increase in LIC and LMIC because of population growth.

Importantly, childhood cancers represent the leading cause of disease-related morbidity and mortality in childhood in HIC, second to accidents as a cause of pediatric death.

J. Mora (✉)
Pediatric Oncology, Pediatric Cancer Center Barcelona (PCCB), Universitat de Barcelona, Barcelona, Spain
e-mail: jaume.mora@sjd.es

G. Chantada
Outreach program, Pediatric Cancer Center Barcelona (PCCB), Universitat de Barcelona, Barcelona, Spain
e-mail: guillermoluis.chantada@sjd.es

L. Krauel (ed.), *Survival Handbook in Pediatric Surgical Oncology*,
https://doi.org/10.1007/978-3-031-65890-7_1

1.3 Outcomes

Age-standardized 5-year survival for children diagnosed with acute lymphocytic leukemia (ALL) in LMICs during 2010–2014 varies between 47.8% (in Ecuador) and 85.7% (in Belarus). The highest survival in ALL in HIC is 95.1% (Finland). Estimates of 5-year survival for all cancers combined broadly range from only 7.4% in LIC to 79.8% in HIC [3].

In LMIC settings, socioeconomic factors influence the diagnostic interval, and delayed diagnosis is typically seen. In addition, even when the diagnosis is timely and the chances of cure are reasonably high, many families in these settings may not accept the proposed treatment or abandon therapy before completion, adding an increased avoidable mortality in these patients. In 2018, the World Health Organization (WHO) set a global survival target of 60% for six index cancers that have greater than 90% survival in HIC [4]. These tumors include ALL, low-grade glioma, retinoblastoma, Burkitt's lymphoma, Hodgkin's lymphoma, and Wilms tumor. It is expected that a million more lives will be saved by the year 2030 [4]. About 89% of the world's children and adolescents (aged 0–19 years) live in LMIC, and they account for 95% of the mortality from cancer in this age group worldwide [3].

1.4 Etiology and Epidemiology

Most childhood cancers arise via stochastic developmental errors compounded by inherited susceptibility [5]. Environmental exposures possibly linked to pediatric cancer are numerous, but most are weak and inconsistent. To date, the only accepted causal agent, albeit under exceptional circumstances (atomic bomb), is ionizing radiation [5].

Germline mutations in cancer-predisposing genes were identified in 8.5% of the children and adolescents with cancer in the largest studies [6]. Family history is commonly used to identify persons with a possible heritable predisposition; however, only 40% of the patients with germline mutations had a family history of cancer. In addition, only half of those had a family history that was consistent with a known cancer predisposition syndrome. On the basis of these observations, family history cannot be the sole indication used to guide genetic testing [6].

Revolutionary advances in next-generation sequencing technology, together with progress in chromatin and stem cell biology, have opened a new era of molecular understanding of childhood cancer. Landmark sequencing studies have demonstrated that the mutational burden is substantially lower than adult cancers [7, 8], whereas fusion genes are more common than in adult cancers, and certain mutations found in pediatric cancers are rare in adult malignancies. The common theme among childhood cancers is that epigenetic dysregulation is central. Furthermore, evidence suggests that many pediatric tumors originate from stem or progenitor cells during particular developmental time windows. It is clear that these cells of origin provide a permissive context for the tumorigenic effects of a genetic or epigenetic hit, which favor self-renewal over differentiation [9]. Thus, the developmental context of cells in which tumorigenic mutations occur and the microenvironment in which they form, both underscore the unique biology of childhood cancer [9].

1.5 Survivors

Cure is not enough, in pediatric cancer care.

With the overall improvement of pediatric cancer survival rates, it has become evident that pediatric cancer survivors are at risk of accelerated physiologic aging [10]. They have a high risk of early mortality from subsequent cancers, cardiac events, and pulmonary conditions. It is typically treatment-specific factors that determine the risk of adverse late effects. Cancer survivors whose treatment included radiation therapy are at risk of secondary neoplasms including cancers of the skin (predominantly basal cell carcinoma), breast, thyroid, bone, and brain. More recently radiation-associated risks for the colon and rectum, kidney, and lung have been documented. Chemotherapeutic drugs are associated with a broad range of potential long-term late effects. Alkylating agents can cause gonadal dysfunction, pulmonary fibrosis, urinary tract abnormalities, renal dysfunction, ototoxicity, and dyslipidemia. Anthracycline antibiotics can induce left ventricular dysfunction, cardiomyopathy, or dysrhythmias. Antimetabolites like methotrexate can cause neurocognitive impairment, leukoencephalopathy, liver dysfunction, renal toxicity, and lower bone mineral density. Corticosteroids are well associated with the development of reduced bone mineral density, osteonecrosis, and cataracts. Epipodophyllotoxins can induce secondary acute myeloid leukemia. Vinca alkaloids induce peripheral sensory and motor neuropathy. Overall, the risk is generally dependent on the cumulative dose, but it also depends on the scheduling and route of administration, as well as the sex and age of the patient.

Surgical procedures performed during diagnosis or treatment of cancer can have long-term effects on health status and quality of life. Examples include amputation and limb-sparing procedures that can affect physical function but also psychological maturation and mental health; eye enucleation, which affects craniofacial development; oophorectomy or orchiectomy, which affects reproduction; cystectomy, which affects bladder or renal function; splenectomy, which affects risk of infection; and neurosurgical procedures that can result in neurocognitive, neuroendocrine, or motor/sensory deficits and in seizures; or spinal cord injury that results in incontinence or sexual dysfunction. Beyond the functional implications of surgery, scarring and disfigurement can also affect the quality of life of survivors. A multidisciplinary approach is mandatory for the management of children with cancer, especially at the time of diagnosis, so extensive and mutilating surgical procedures are avoided when possible.

References

1. Mora J. What is a pediatric tumor? Clin Oncol Adolesc Young Adults. 2012;2:7–15.
2. Atun R, et al. Sustainable care for children with cancer: a Lancet Oncology Commission. Lancet Oncol. 2020;21(4):e185–224.
3. Rodriguez-Galindo C, et al. Toward the cure of all children with cancer through collaborative efforts: pediatric oncology as a global challenge. J Clin Oncol. 2015;33:3065–73.
4. https://www.who.int/publications/i/item/9789240025271
5. Greaves M. A causal mechanism for childhood acute lymphoblastic leukaemia. Nat Rev Cancer. 2018;18(8):471–84.
6. Zhang J, et al. Germline mutations in predisposition genes in pediatric cancer. N Engl J Med. 2015;373:2336–46.
7. Gröbner SN, et al. The landscape of genomic alterations across childhood cancers. Nature. 2018;555:321–7.
8. Ma X, et al. Pan-cancer genome and transcriptome analyses of 1,699 paediatric leukaemias and solid tumours. Nature. 2018;555:371–6.
9. Filbin M, Monje M. Developmental origins and emerging therapeutic opportunities for childhood cancer. Nat Med. 2019;25(3):367–76.
10. Robison LL, Hudson MM. Survivors of childhood and adolescent cancer: life-long risks and responsibilities. Nat Rev Cancer. 2014;14:61–70.

The Importance of Tumor Board and the Role of the Surgeon

2

Lucas Krauel and Rosalia Carrasco Torrents

2.1 Introduction

Pediatric surgical oncology is a complex and challenging field that requires a multidisciplinary approach. The care of children with cancer involves a range of healthcare professionals, including surgeons, oncologists, radiation therapists, nurses, and social workers. To provide the best possible care for these patients, it is essential to have a coordinated and collaborative approach to their management. Tumor boards are critical in this regard, a unique opportunity to bring together healthcare professionals from different specialties to discuss all aspects of management including diagnosis, prognosis, and treatment, of each individual patient.

2.2 Definition of Tumor Board

A tumor board is a multidisciplinary team of healthcare professionals who meet regularly to discuss all aspects of each individual cancer patient with the aim to achieve a unique and common plan of management. The goal of the tumor board is to ensure that patients receive the most appropriate and effective management for their cancer, based on a comprehensive and individualized evaluation of their medical history, imaging studies, pathology reports, biological studies, and other tests. Tumor boards are usually led by a medical oncologist, radiation oncologist, or surgeon and include other healthcare professionals such as radiologists; pathologists; rehabilitators; palliative and quality-of-care specialists; molecular biologists; radiation oncologists; researchers; consultants in nephrology, neurology, and dermatology; nurses; and others.

2.3 Importance of Tumor Board in Pediatric Surgical Oncology

In pediatric surgical oncology, tumor boards play a key role in the management of children with cancer. Because pediatric cancers are rare and complex, it is critically important to have a coordinated approach to their management, involving healthcare professionals with specialized knowledge and expertise in this field. Tumor boards bring together these experts to discuss individual cases and develop a comprehensive treatment plan that takes into account the unique needs and circumstances of each patient.

One of the key benefits of tumor boards is that they facilitate communication and collabo-

L. Krauel (✉) · R. C. Torrents
Pediatric Surgical Oncology, Pediatric Surgery Department, Pediatric Cancer Center Barcelona (PCCB), SJD Barcelona Children's Hospital, Universitat de Barcelona, Barcelona, Spain
e-mail: lucas.krauel@sjd.es; rosalia.carrasco@sjd.es

L. Krauel (ed.), *Survival Handbook in Pediatric Surgical Oncology*,
https://doi.org/10.1007/978-3-031-65890-7_2

ration among healthcare professionals from different specialties. By working together to review diagnostic information and develop a treatment plan, tumor boards ensure that all aspects of a patient's care are coordinated and consistent. This is particularly important in pediatric surgical oncology, where children often require surgery, chemotherapy, immunotherapy, and radiation therapy, as well as supportive care for side effects and other complications of treatment.

By bringing together healthcare professionals with different areas of expertise, tumor boards ensure that all treatment options are considered and that the elected treatment is tailored to the individual patient's needs and circumstances.

Tumor boards can help enroll patients in most suitable clinical trials when appropriate. Clinical trials are essential for advancing the understanding and treatment of pediatric cancers, but they require careful evaluation and selection of patients based on their medical history, disease characteristics, and other factors. Tumor boards help to identify patients who may be eligible for clinical trials and ensure that they are enrolled at the right time during the course of the disease.

Finally, tumor boards can play an important role in supporting families and caregivers of children with cancer. By bringing together healthcare professionals from different specialties, tumor boards allow for a coordinated and compassionate approach to the care of children with cancer. This can help to alleviate some of the stress and anxiety that families and caregivers may experience during this difficult time.

Tumor boards should have a designated secretary who keeps record of all the discussions held and what is the final consensus reached. It is important to note that the tumor board should be open to all specialists (oncology and non-oncology related) in order to discuss challenging cases that might raise the question as to whether a patient has an oncologic process.

2.4 Conclusion

Tumor boards are an essential tool in the management of children with cancer. By bringing together healthcare professionals from different specialties, tumor boards can ensure that patients receive the most appropriate and effective treatment for their cancer, tailored to their individual needs and circumstances. Tumor boards facilitate communication and collaboration among healthcare professionals, support enrollment in clinical trials, and provide compassionate care to families and caregivers. As such, tumor boards are a critical component of pediatric surgical oncology and thus are an integral part of the surgeon's commitment to the patients.

3 Pediatric Oncology for Surgeons: Principles of Chemotherapy and Radiotherapy

Maite Gorostegui and JI Toscas

3.1 Introduction

Chemotherapy, surgery, and radiotherapy have improved outcomes of childhood cancer over the last decades. To date, the 5-year survival is 80% for the majority of children and adolescents in high-income countries. Despite this, the prognosis of many high-risk diseases remains dismal. The increased understanding of the biology of cancer has allowed the addition of immunotherapy and targeted therapies for some entities [1].

For surgeons it is important to know the principles of these therapies, the implications for surgical decision-making, and the pre- and postoperative care [2].

Radiotherapy uses high-energy radiation to damage DNA and destroy cancer cells. Although its use has been decreasing over time, it plays a crucial role in different settings, especially as consolidation treatment of several solid malignancies.

Fortunately, the great technological development witnessed in the last two decades has drastically transformed the way it is delivered. Current treatment modalities allow to better conform the dose to the tumor target volume, while significantly reducing the dose received by nearby healthy tissues. Taking into account the rise in the number of long-term survivors and the possibility of experiencing long-term side effects, dose reduction in healthy tissues is particularly relevant.

3.2 Chemotherapy/Targeted Therapy Overview

Chemo drugs target normal and cancer cells, interfering with the process of cell proliferation in different ways such as the induction of DNA breaks, blocking DNA synthesis, affecting microtubules, etc. [3]

Since the first complete remission in children with acute lymphoblastic leukemia was reported in the late 1940s, chemo agents have become one of the major pillars of cancer treatment in children. To overcome chemoresistance, conventional chemotherapy is given as a combination that may include alkylating agents, antimetabolites, antibiotics, topoisomerase inhibitors, mitotic inhibitors, and corticosteroids.

More recent understanding of tumor behavior and molecular tumor characteristics has allowed us to target unique genetic features of patients' tumors. Although this strategy has more application in adults, there is also increasing evidence in specific pediatric tumors.

M. Gorostegui (✉)
Pediatric Oncology Department, Pediatric Cancer Center Barcelona (PCCB), SJD Barcelona Children's Hospital, Universitat de Barcelona, Barcelona, Spain
e-mail: maite.gorostegui@sjd.es

JI. Toscas
Radiotherapy Department, Teknon Oncologic Institute, Barcelona, Spain

L. Krauel (ed.), *Survival Handbook in Pediatric Surgical Oncology*,
https://doi.org/10.1007/978-3-031-65890-7_3

Chemotherapy agents and common adverse effects [5]

L-Asparaginase/PEG-ASP/ Erwinase	Transaminitis, pancreatitis, glucose intolerance, coagulopathy
Bleomycin	Nausea/vomiting, fever, pneumonitis/pulmonary fibrosis, stomatitis, skin rash
Carboplatin and cisplatin	Nausea/vomiting, allergic reactions/anaphylactic shock, kidney failure, myelosuppression, ototoxicity
Cyclophosphamide	Nausea/vomiting, myelosuppression (after weeks), pulmonary fibrosis, stomatitis, hemorrhagic cystitis
Cytarabine (Ara-C)	Nausea/vomiting, myelosuppression, conjunctivitis, mucositis, ataxia
Dactinomycin	Nausea/vomiting, extravasation injury, myelosuppression, mucositis
Doxorubicin, daunorubicin, idarubicin	Nausea/vomiting, cardiotoxicity, red-colored urine, extravasation injury, myelosuppression, dermatitis
Etoposide	Nausea/vomiting, hypotension, skin rash
Ifosfamide	Nausea/vomiting, hemorrhagic cystitis (prevent with mesna), renal toxicity, myelosuppression, encephalopathy, SIADH[a]
6-Mercaptopurine	Myelosuppression, hepatitis
Methotrexate	Mucositis, nephrotoxicity, hepatitis, neurotoxicity
Corticosteroids	Cushing syndrome, diabetes, hypertension, osteoporosis, avascular necrosis femoral head, behavioral changes, cataracts
Irinotecan	Diarrhea, cholinergic syndrome
Temozolomide	Nausea/vomiting, myelosuppression with late onset (3 weeks after)
Vincristine	Constipation, peripheral neuropathy, jaw pain, ileus, SIADH

[a] Syndrome of inappropriate antidiuretic hormone secretion

Chemotherapy and precision oncology agents can be administered before surgery and/or radiation as a neoadjuvant or after local control as an adjuvant therapy. In the neoadjuvant setting, chemotherapy classically has been used to decrease the tumor bulk and facilitate the surgery. With the same objective, biological therapies are currently in use, e.g., NTRK inhibitors in large infantile fibrosarcoma, ALK inhibitors in malignant peritoneal mesothelioma, or some cases of inflammatory myofibroblastic tumors.

As a rule, any neoadjuvant strategy has the potential to impair wound healing and infection risk. Although no evidence-based guidelines exist, pediatric surgeons need to be aware of timing considerations; the concern of wound complications needs to be balanced against the impact of prolonged oncological therapy cessation on treatment efficacy (see checklist below).

A list of secondary effects—acute and long term—can follow chemo administration. For surgeons, acute effects during the neutropenic phase, usually 7–14 days after the initiation of chemotherapy, are of utmost importance; mucositis, enterocolitis, anal fissures with secondary perianal abscess, and invasive fungal infection can become evident during the neutrophils recovery.

Pancreatitis is typically associated with asparaginase use. It seems to be more related to genetic predisposition than to the accumulated dose [4].

Hemorrhagic cystitis can be secondary to ifosfamide and cyclophosphamide; however, currently, since these drugs are given with mesna and aggressive hydration, this is rarely seen. Nowadays, hemorrhagic cystitis is more often seen in patients undergoing stem cell transplantation due to multifactorial risks, after viral infection (BK virus) or secondary to radiation.

Children undergoing multimodal treatment may also experience potential complications that necessitate surgical management. These may include severe neutropenic enterocolitis and perforations resulting from chemotherapy, as well as pneumothorax associated with targeted therapies such as pazopanib. Maintaining a heightened level of suspicion is crucial for promptly detecting these less common complications.

3.3 Advances in Radiotherapy Technology for Pediatric Patients

Progress in clinical radiotherapy has been strongly related to technical developments leading to more precise tumor irradiation. After the introduction of three-dimensional conformal radiotherapy, based on computed tomography that allowed the delimitation of the target volumes, and the organs to be spared, the next step was the introduction of high-precision techniques, which today are the standard of care for many pediatric tumors [6].

Intensity-Modulated-Radiation Therapy (IMRT) Allows the possibility to adapt the dose distributions to the geometric shape of anatomic structures and modulates intensity to deliver the dose to the clinical target and spare healthy organs [7].

Volumetric Modulated Arc Therapy (VMAT) Implies a system that rotates around the patient, while the radiation beam is shaped and modulated to conform closely to the shape of the tumor. Allows for shorter treatment delivery times compared with conventional techniques [8].

Proton Therapy Protons are positively charged particles with a biological effectiveness roughly similar to high-energy photons. However, unlike photons, proton beams have a finite range in tissue that eliminates the exit dose for each radiation beam and greatly reduces it in the overlying tissues. This unique physical characteristic of protons provides a superior dose distribution, compared to photons, and an optimal target conformation that delivers a lower dose to the non-target tissues nearby. This is what makes proton therapy so appealing in pediatric RT.

There are numerous pediatric tumor locations in which, even though high doses are successfully delivered with conventional photon techniques, the caveat is a high risk of severe late effects (e.g., growth and developmental, endocrinological and fertility, neuropsychological, and treatment-induced second cancers) that may significantly worsen the quality of life of the cured children [6, 9, 10].

The high cost of building proton therapy facilities in the twentieth century and the absence of commercially available treatment units worldwide have limited the indications and clinical research in the early times. By the end of the 1990s the Children's Oncology Group accepted for the first time proton therapy in children with rhabdomyosarcomas included in their prospective trial D9602. Nowadays, proton therapy is accepted, when available, as the primary indication for most pediatric solid tumors, particularly central nervous system tumors [10]. Proton therapy is presently linked to a significant reduction in severe late effects such as neuroendocrine, cochlear dose-related problems, cardiologic (e.g., abnormal Q waves and impaired maximum cardiac index), pulmonary (e.g., restrictive lung disease), esophageal (structures), and second cancers [11, 12].

3.3.1 Radiation Therapy Treatment: Workflow

Each patient should be evaluated by a multidisciplinary tumor board to provide personalized, comprehensive, and evidence-based treatment recommendations. As a pre-treatment phase, patients undergo a planning CT scan in a reproducible position. The images obtained can be matched with preoperative imaging to precisely define the location of the tumor. After identifying the target volume and organs at risk (OARs), radiation oncologists, medical physicists, and dosimetrists create a personalized treatment plan based on the imaging data and tumor characteristics (Fig. 3.1).

Evidence-based radiation dose-volume guidelines for normal tissue constraints have been proposed by the PENTEC (Pediatric Normal Tissue Effects in the Clinic) research project [13].

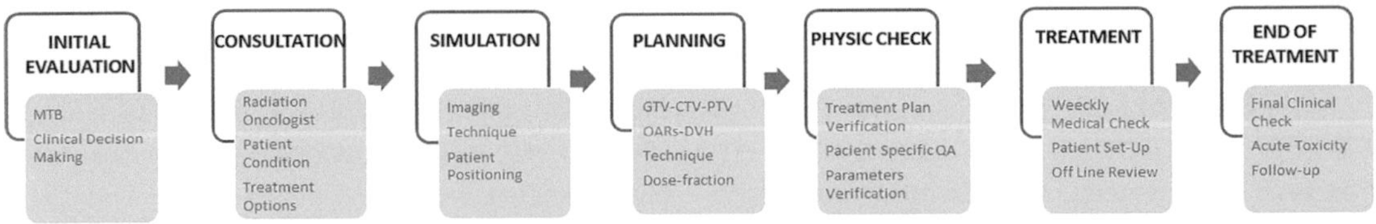

Fig. 3.1 Workflow radiation treatment process. *MTB* multidisciplinary tumor board, *GTV* gross tumor volume, *CTV* clinical tumor volume, *PTV* planning treatment volume, *OARs* organs at risk, *DVH* dose-volume histogram, *QA* quality assurance

Be aware of the following definitions represented in Fig. 3.2:

- **Gross Tumor Volume (GTV)**: The visible tumor identified through imaging. In post-surgery treatment, a virtual GTV should be created based on preoperative imaging.
- **Clinical Tumor Volume (CTV)**: This is the volume that contains the GTV with an additional margin of around (5–10 mm), to take into account the microscopic tumor spread.
- **Planning Target Volume (PTV)**: This is the final volume for treatment planning. Includes an additional margin around the CTV (5–10 mm), to account for organ movement and patient set-up errors.
- **Dose-Volume Histogram (DVH)**: This is a quantitative graphical representation of dose distribution vs. volume in the target and OARs. It is an essential element in the planning process since through detailed analysis it makes it possible to identify areas where the dose exceeds the tolerance limits. This is used to evaluate the possible complications related to the treatment.

Surgeon's Checklist

1. No signs of infection and counts recovery are key. Usually 2–3 weeks after chemo (be aware that platins often need more time for platelets recovery).

If your patient is receiving target therapy, it is recommended:

1. TKIs (tyrosine kinase inhibitors) (larotrectinib, regorafenib, etc.): holding 1 week preoperative and 2 weeks postoperative (*variations depending on the drug's half-life*).
2. VEGFR inhibitors (bevacizumab): holding 4 weeks preoperative and 4 weeks postoperative (until the surgical wound is healed).
3. mTOR inhibitors (rapamycin, everolimus, tacrolimus): dose reductions are effective (transplant setting). Additionally consider preoperative antibiotics and the use of closed suction drains.
4. AlK inhibitors (crizotinib, alectinib, lorlatinib, etc.): can be restarted early after surgery. The discontinuation of this therapy before surgery usually is due to potential interactions with anesthetics during surgery.

During surgery think about the next treatment step for your patient:

1. Whenever possible a maximum resection of the tumor should be performed.
2. Surgical clips are needed as reference points during treatment planning, especially in cases where complete surgery has not been feasible, and the residual tumor volume must be boosted.
3. Generally, the greater the residual disease, the more radiation dose is needed for local control.

Keep a high index of suspicion for the following agents and potential complications not operative-related:

1. L-Asparaginase: pancreatitis.
2. High-dose cyclophosphamide, ifosfamide, and busulfan: hemorrhagic cystitis.
3. Bevacizumab: gastrointestinal perforation.
4. Regorafenib: colonic perforation.
5. Pazopanib: spontaneous pneumothorax.

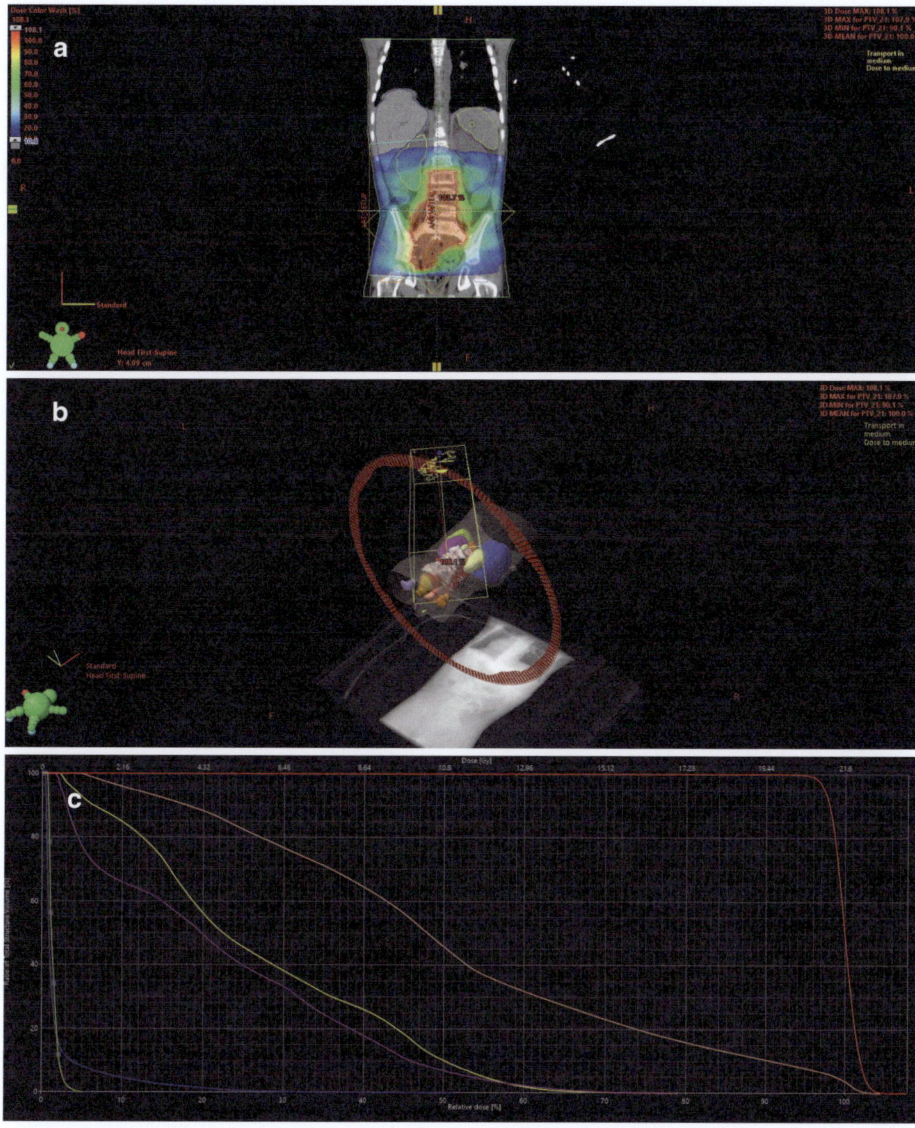

Fig. 3.2 Treatment plan showing 95% isodose line coverage PTV (red), coronal image. Liver (blue); left kidney (magenta); right kidney (yellow); spleen (green) (**a**). Volumetric modulated arc therapy (VMAT) plans 3D reconstruction view (**b**). Dose-volume histogram (DVH): bin dose along the horizontal axis and organ volume on the vertical (**c**)

References

1. Tydings C, Kim A. Technology and precision therapy delivery in childhood cancer. Curr Opin Pediatr. 2020;32(1):1–6.
2. Harris CJ, Waters AM, Tracy ET, Christison-Lagay E, Baertshiger RM, Ehrlich P, Abdessalam S, Aldrink JH, Rhee DS, Dasgupta R, Rodeberg DA, Lautz TB. Precision oncology: a primer for pediatric surgeons from the APSA Cancer Committee. J Pediatr Surg. 2020;55(9):1706–13.
3. Bo L, Wang Y, Li Y, Wurpel JND, Huang Z, Chen ZS. The battlefield of chemotherapy in pediatric cancers. Cancers (Basel). 2023;15(7):1963.
4. De Campos Vieira S, Chui Chan H, Cox S, et al. International Society of Pediatric Surgical Oncology (IPSO) surgical practice guidelines. Ecancermedicalscience. 2022;16:1356.
5. Flosi T, D'Augustine S. Tarascon pediatric inpatient pocketbook. Jones & Bartlett Learning; 2016.

6. Hua CH, Mascia AE, Seravalli E, et al. Advances in radiotherapy technology for pediatric cancer patients and roles of medical physicists: COG and SIOP Europe perspectives. Pediatr Blood Cancer. 2021;68(Suppl2):e28344.
7. Kalapurakal JA, Zhang Y, Kepka A, et al. Cardiac-sparing whole lung IMRT in children with lung metástasis. Int J Radiat Oncol Biol Phys. 2013;85(3):761–7.
8. Fogliata A, Bergström S, Cafaro I, et al. Cranio-spinal irradiation with volumetric modulated arc therapy: a multi-institutional treatment experience. Radiother Oncol. 2011;99:79–85.
9. Coltin H, Pequeno P, Liu N, et al. The burden of surviving childhood medulloblastoma: a population-based, matched cohort study in Ontario, Canada. J Clin Oncol. 2023;41:2372–82.
10. Indelicato DJ, Merchant T, Laperriere N, et al. Consensus report from the Stockholm Pediatric Proton Therapy Conference. Int J Radiat Oncol Biol Phys. 2016;96:387–92.
11. Eaton BR, Esiashvili N, Kim S, et al. Clinical outcomes among children with standard-risk medulloblastoma treated with proton and photon radiation therapy: a comparison of disease control and overall survival. Int J Radiat Oncol Biol Phys. 2016;94:133–8.
12. Yock TI, Yeap BY, Ebb DH, et al. Long-term toxic effects of proton radiotherapy for paediatric medulloblastoma: a phase 2 single-arm study. Lancet Oncol. 2016;17:287–98.
13. Constine LS, Ronckers CM, Hua CH, et al. Pediatric normal tissue effects in clinic (PENTEC): an international collaboration to analyze normal tissue radiation dose-volume response relationships for pediatric cancer patients. Clin Oncol (R Coll Radiol). 2019;32(3):199–207.

Radiology in Pediatric Cancer

4

Enrique Ladera Gonzalez and Ignasi Barber

4.1 Introduction

The diagnostic and therapeutic approach to childhood oncological pathology is highly complex and delicate, and medical imaging plays a paramount role. In addition, image-guided interventional radiology has gained relevance in the management of these patients.

Choosing the best imaging technique at any given time of the process is difficult, and coordination between pediatricians, surgeons, and radiologists is vital for patient management and resource optimization [1]. Regarding imaging, X-rays, ultrasounds, computed tomography, and MRI are common techniques, but we cannot leave behind other techniques such as fluoroscopy or nuclear medicine studies (scintigraphy, positron emission tomography-computed tomography (PET-CT), PET-MRI). Each of these studies will have a different use in management, as explained below.

E. L. Gonzalez (✉)
Radiology Department, Interventional Radiology, Pediatric Cancer Center Barcelona (PCCB), SJD Barcelona Children's Hospital, Universitat de Barcelona, Barcelona, Spain
e-mail: enrique.ladera@sjd.es

I. Barber
Radiology Department, Pediatric Cancer Center Barcelona (PCCB), SJD Barcelona Children's Hospital, Universitat de Barcelona, Barcelona, Spain
e-mail: ignacio.barber@sjd.es

4.2 Radiology and Diagnosis

When an oncological debut takes place, two clinical needs arise: (1) identify the lesion, its location and size, and involvement of neighboring structures, and (2) identify subclinical metastatic lesions. Both objectives must be met quickly, to reduce decision-making time and start the proper treatment.

X-ray is useful in locating chest lesions or bone lesions, and ultrasound is powerful in identifying soft tissue lesions. Both techniques are accessible and easy to perform at the time of diagnosis. These techniques might also be the best choice to guide biopsies or placement of vascular catheters.

Once the lesion has been identified, cross-sectional imaging using CT or MRI will offer a detailed study of the entire tumor volume. Both techniques are useful in defining the margins of the lesions, their local extension, and, to some extent, their tissular characteristics (Fig. 4.1). This amount of data, called tissue radiomics will allow not only to make a differential diagnosis based on imaging alone but also to provide information regarding the best area for sample biopsy [2].

Although CT or MRI might not be available at the time of presentation, it is recommended to perform these studies before surgery or other invasive processes on the tumor.

In the following quadrant, we see each technique and its pros and cons (Table 4.1).

L. Krauel (ed.), *Survival Handbook in Pediatric Surgical Oncology*,
https://doi.org/10.1007/978-3-031-65890-7_4

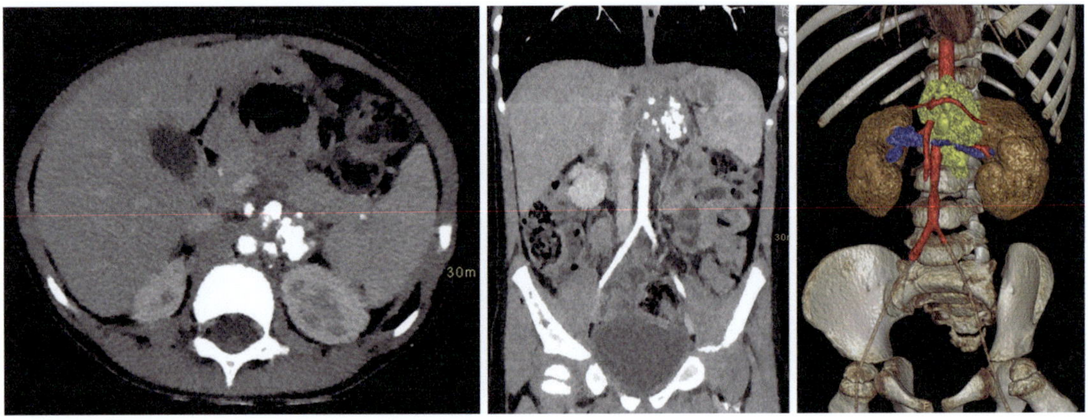

Fig. 4.1 Contrast abdominal CT axial and coronal images and 3D reconstruction: retroperitoneal calcified lesion can be assessed and its relationships with retroperitoneal vessels

Table 4.1 Pros and cons of radiological techniques

Technique	X-ray	Ultrasound	CT	MRI
Utility	Immediate, useful in the bone and lungs	Immediate, useful in soft tissue lesions	Fastk, easy to perform, 3D image, high spatial resolution, good vascular assessment	High spatial resolution Limited specificity, provides information about the tumor tissue, no radiation
Cons	No volumetric information	Limited volumetric information, lower specificity in large lesions	Radiation, usually provides limited tissular information IV iodine contrast	Usually not available, requires anesthesia, poor vascular assessment
In surgery	On-site use	On-site use	3D planning	3D planning

For the disease extension study, the technique depends on the type of tumor and the most common location of metastasis. All organs likely to contain metastases must be studied. Techniques that include the entire organism are whole-body MRI (WB-MRI), PET-CT, bone scan or body CT. Segmented studies can also be performed, for example, abdominal MRI + chest CT, in case the possible metastases are located in the lungs. These tests should be performed promptly, preferably after knowing the pathological diagnosis.

4.3 Image-Assisted Process

The image takes on a special role for the surgeon when it allows guiding minimally invasive procedures. For this, real-time techniques (fluoroscopy and ultrasound) are useful, allowing for better eye-hand correlation. In certain cases it can be complemented with reconstructions performed with CT, MRI, or nuclear medicine studies, and fused images might be generated.

4.3.1 Needle Location

The use of ultrasound is very useful (Fig. 4.2) to guide needles in soft tissues, for example, for vascular access, or biopsy needles fine needle aspiration cytology (FNAC) or biopsy aspiration gun (BAG). Trained personnel and multidisciplinary teamwork among interventional radiologists and surgeons is recommended.

In other occasions, ultrasound might be able to identify lesions that are difficult to assess by the eye. The radiologist may leave one or more markers in the lesion to facilitate surgical removal. Widely used markers are harpoons or material injected into the injury, such as dyes (blue) or radioisotopes (which are then detected with a handheld gamma camera).

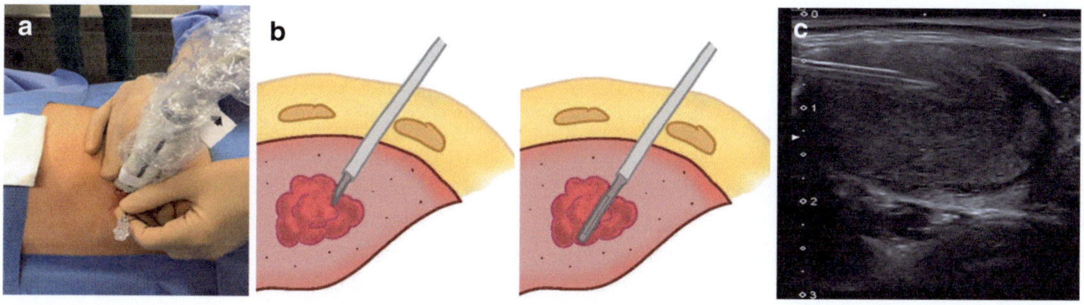

Fig. 4.2 (**a**) Ultrasound-guided biopsy through a coaxial needle. (**b**) Drawings of an ultrasound-guided biopsy. (**c**) Ultrasound image where a needle biopsying a thyroid mass can be seen

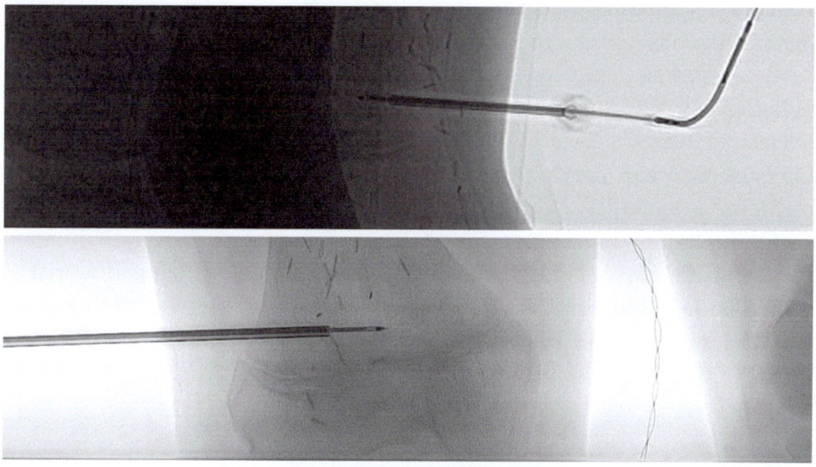

Fig. 4.3 Radiology guidance of a percutaneous cryoablation of a parosteal osteosarcoma

4.3.2 Therapeutic Imaging-Guided Intervention

Imaging techniques are also useful to guide therapeutic procedures including cryotherapy or cryoablation, radioablation or chemoembolization (using endovascular interventional techniques) (Fig. 4.3).

4.4 Radiology in the Follow-Up

As in the initial assessment, imaging plays a key role in the posttreatment reassessment. It is recommended to reevaluate after the use of neoadjuvant chemotherapy treatment, to plan the surgery of the lesion. At this point, radiomics of the lesion is very important as it provides data on posttreatment necrosis, which is a prognostic factor [2]. Of course, it will also identify areas of liquefaction, bleeding, or size variations that the surgeon will need to take into account. In cases in which the lesion is resistant to treatment, that is, it continues to grow despite therapy, post-neoadjuvant reassessment may lead to reconsidering the surgery.

It is recommended to perform the same imaging technique that was used for initial evaluation, making both images and data sets comparable.

After surgical treatment, it is crucial to assess whether any tumor remnants are present in the surgical bed or the area previously occupied by the tumor. It should be noted that the surgery itself, along with postsurgical devices in the patient (such as osteosynthesis materials, hemostatic agents, etc.), as well as potential postsurgical hematomas or seromas, can complicate this assessment. Therefore, it is generally advisable to delay imaging until after the initial postsurgical period, unless an acute complication is suspected [3].

Once the treatment has been completed, the patient will require periodic imaging control to detect local or metastatic recurrence. Ultrasound of the abdomen or soft tissues and plain film of the chest are usually good imaging techniques for long-term follow-up. MRI is also useful given its absence of radiation burden and high sensitivity for local relapse detection on lesions throughout the body [4].

4.5 Conclusions

Pediatric oncology is rare, very varied, and complex, and good coordination between team members, including oncologists, surgeons, and radiologists, is paramount. Radiologist and nuclear medicine specialists at each center are the ones who can provide the best information regarding availability and appropriateness criteria for the different imaging techniques.

The usefulness of each imaging technique should be individualized. As general guidelines, we can summarize the following key points:

- In the initial diagnosis, X-ray and ultrasound will give an initial approach, and cross-sectional imaging using CT or MR is the second step. Disease extension evaluation is performed with separate techniques (abdominal ultrasound + chest CT), selected imaging, as chest CT only, or whole-body imaging (usually PET-CT) (Fig. 4.4).
- Imaging is also useful to guide sample biopsies or surgical procedures.
- In the posttreatment follow-up imaging should consider both local control and the appearance of distant metastasis.

Surgeon's Checklist

1. Check with the radiology team to ascertain the most appropriate imaging technique for each unique case and situation.
2. When initially approaching a mass, consider utilizing low-risk and cost-effective techniques, such as X-ray (for bone and chest) or ultrasound (for soft tissue).

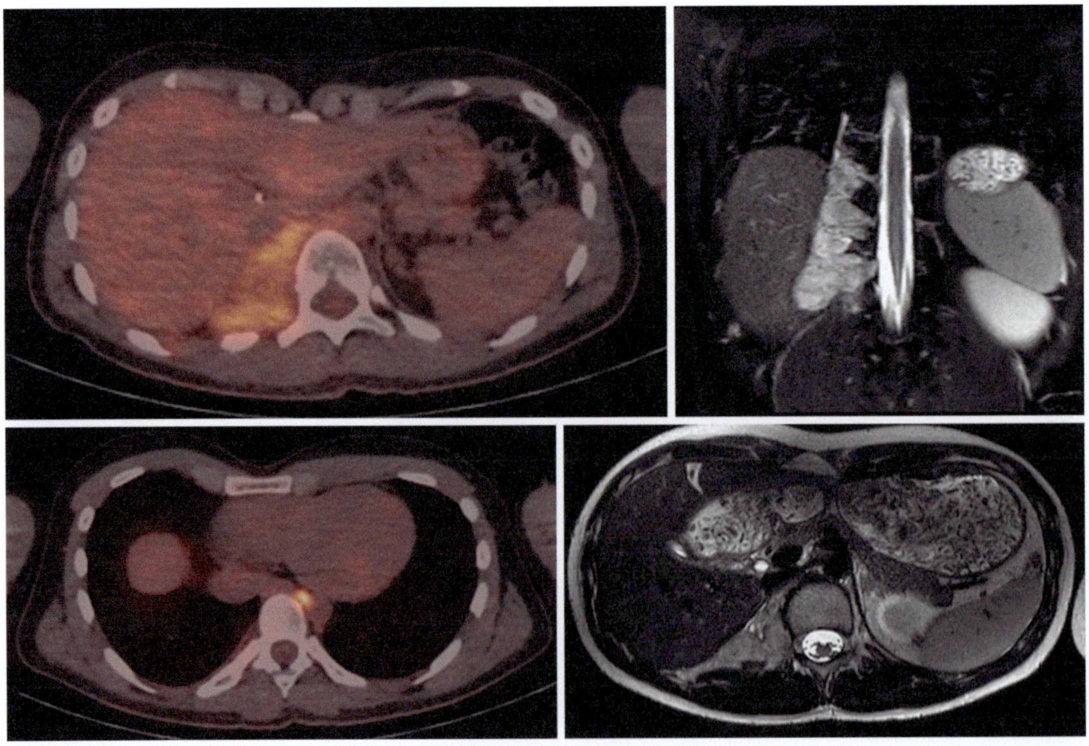

Fig. 4.4 PET-CT and MRI imaging of a paravertebral neuroblastoma

3. Utilize cross-sectional imaging, such as CT or MRI, to assess the entire volume of the lesion. Ideally, perform this before invasive techniques like biopsies.
4. Employ whole-body imaging to assess potential metastasis, utilizing methods like whole-body MRI, PET-CT, or a combination of techniques such as abdominal ultrasound and chest CT.
5. Use real-time imaging (ultrasound, fluoroscopy) to guide minimally invasive procedures, including biopsies or therapeutic interventions. Consider leaving markers during this process to aid surgeons in locating specific areas during surgery.
6. During surgical planning, discuss with your radiology team all the information you need to control the morphology and anatomy of the lesion. If required, perform specific techniques such as angio-CT, local MRI, ultrasound, or Doppler ultrasound to gather essential information.
7. During follow-up, ensure to check the local area and assess the possibility of metastasis. Whole-body images and cost-effective imaging methods prove to be valuable.

References

1. Aguado A. Role of interventional radiology in pediatric cancer patients. Curr Oncol Rep. 2022;24(12):1731–40. https://doi.org/10.1007/s11912-022-01320-1. Epub 2022 Sep 3.
2. Davendralingam N, Sebire NJ, Arthurs OJ, Shelmerdine SC. Artificial intelligence in paediatric radiology: future opportunities. Br J Radiol. 2021;94(1117):20200975. https://doi.org/10.1259/bjr.20200975. Epub 2020 Sep 17.
3. Handa A, Nozaki T, Makidono A, Okabe T, Morita Y, Fujita K, Matsusako M, Kono T, Kurihara Y, Hasegawa D, Kumamoto T, Ogawa C, Yuza Y, Manabe A. Pediatric oncologic emergencies: clinical and imaging review for pediatricians. Pediatr Int. 2019;61(2):122–39. https://doi.org/10.1111/ped.13755. Epub 2019 Feb 7.
4. Guimarães MD, Noschang J, Teixeira SR, Santos MK, Lederman HM, Tostes V, Kundra V, Oliveira AD, Hochhegger B, Marchiori E. Whole-body MRI in pediatric patients with cancer. Cancer Imaging. 2017;17(1):6. https://doi.org/10.1186/s40644-017-0107-7.

Anesthesia in Pediatric Cancer

5

Alicia Chamizo and Mario Cuesta Argos

5.1 Introduction

Pediatric anesthesia differs in important ways from anesthesia for adults, and it is worldwide recognized as a specific area of expertise. Moreover, anesthesia and pain management in pediatric cancer represent a higher challenge for pediatric anesthesiologists.

Anesthesiologists treating patients with cancer have to actively interact with oncological surgeons and oncologists. This is important not only for the outcome of the act of surgery itself but also for preoperative and postoperative issues. It is advisable that anesthesiologists work hand in hand with the multidisciplinary treating team.

In this chapter, we will discuss the general principles of preanesthesia preparation, induction, maintenance of general anesthesia, emergence from anesthesia, and anesthetic emergencies for children with cancer undergoing surgery. We have also provided subsections with tips and tricks for the most common surgical oncology procedures, along with comments on alternative medicines in the management of pain for children with cancer.

5.2 Preoperative Evaluation

The objective is to obtain relevant clinical information that will help during the surgical processes of a patient undergoing cancer treatment. Furthermore, close contact with the child and his family will increase trust and decrease anxiety.

5.2.1 Anamnesis

Regarding the anesthetic history, the patient's health status is assessed using the American Society of Anesthesiologists (ASA) scale (Table 5.1). The ASA scale does not provide

Table 5.1 ASA scale of preoperative health status

ASA	Definition
1	Healthy person
2	Mild systemic disease
3	Severe systemic disease
4	Severe systemic disease that is a constant threat to life
5	A moribund person who is not expected to survive without the operation
6	A declared brain-dead person whose organs are being removed for donor purposes

A. Chamizo (✉)
Pediatric Anesthesia Department, Pediatric Cancer Center Barcelona (PCCB), SJD Barcelona Children's Hospital, Universitat de Barcelona, Barcelona, Spain
e-mail: alicia.chamizo@sjd.es

M. C. Argos
Pediatric Surgical Oncology, Pediatric Surgery Department, Pediatric Cancer Center Barcelona (PCCB), SJD Barcelona Children's Hospital, Universitat de Barcelona, Barcelona, Spain
e-mail: mario.cuesta@sjd.es

L. Krauel (ed.), *Survival Handbook in Pediatric Surgical Oncology*,
https://doi.org/10.1007/978-3-031-65890-7_5

information on the surgical anesthetic risk, for which there are other specific scales.

Other important anamnesis parameters to take into consideration are:

- Medical, surgical, and family history.
- Complications that have occurred in previous surgical procedures.
- Allergies or medications. Children with cancer often take regular medications that may cause reactions and/or synergisms with anesthetic drugs.
- Small details such as a moving tooth.

5.2.2 Physical Examination

5.2.2.1 Upper Airway

Related Problems

- Syndromes that involve **craniofacial malformations**.
- **Tumor location** involving the tongue, neck, or cervical region.

Anesthetics Measures

- It is essential to prepare in advance all the necessary tools to successfully perform airway intubation.
  - The essential materials that should be available are fibrolaryngoscope, pediatric fibrobronchoscopy, and tracheostomy set.
  - If the airway is really difficult, it is advisable to request the support of the otorhinolaryngology team and to suggest to the family the possibility of performing a regular tracheostomy prior to surgery.

5.2.2.2 Respiratory

Related Problems

- **Infection** is the most common cause of acute respiratory failure in children.
  - Increased risk due to immunosuppression and neutropenia in cancer patients.
  - Tenfold increase risk of bronchospasm or laryngospasm.
- Children with **asthma** have a higher risk of bronchospasm, hypercarbia, and acidosis.
- Oncology patients may have associated respiratory problems due to the **disease itself** or the treatments received.
  - Patients with leukemia often have pulmonary infiltrates that resemble pneumonitis.
  - Cardiogenic pulmonary edema may occur after treatment with anthracyclines like doxorubicin.

Anesthetics Measures

- For respiratory infections: if possible, surgery should be delayed for several weeks.
- For asthma: preventive bronchodilator or steroid treatments for 3–5 days before surgery are recommended.
- The risk of severe respiratory complications makes it necessary to consider ventilatory support in the postoperative period with pediatric intensive care unit (PICU) admission.

5.2.2.3 Cardiac

Related Problems

- Cardiac dysfunction in children with cancer can be caused by chemotherapeutic agents like anthracyclines or radiotherapy to the mediastinum.

Anesthetics Measures

- A complete cardiac evaluation should be performed before surgery with electrocardiogram (EKG) and echocardiogram as the most appropriate tests to evaluate noninvasively the heart function [1].

5.2.2.4 Renal and Electrolytes

Related Problems

- Renal and electrolyte disorders in oncological patients may be related to chemotherapeutic agents such as cyclophosphamide, platins, ifosfamide, or methotrexate. Radiotherapy and antibiotics like aminoglycosides or amphotericin can alter electrolyte balance.
- Leukemias and lymphomas are associated with hyperuricemia.

- Patients with Wilms tumor (WT) may have hypertension because of renin secretion.
- Obstructive nephropathy may occur because of external compression by the tumor.
- **Tumor lysis syndrome** is defined by the coexistence of hyperuricemia, hyperkalemia, hypocalcemia, hyperphosphatemia, and renal insufficiency [1–3].

Anesthetics Measures

- In the preoperative blood test, it is advisable to include renal function tests including serum levels of electrolytes and creatinine.
- **Tumor lysis syndrome**: it must be corrected before surgery. It requires close control of potassium with alkalization of urine, diuresis, allopurinol, and calcium supplementation. If dialysis is required, it should be performed 24 h before surgery to achieve the best level of electrolytes and volemia.

5.2.2.5 Metabolic

Related Problems

- Cancer patients often suffer from malnutrition and cachexia of widely varying causes. The drug-free proportions can be modified under these conditions thus increasing the chances of drug-related toxicity.
- Patients with hypopituitarism like craniopharyngiomas should be compensated first with cortisol and thyroxine before operation.
- Many tumors can present with vomiting and diarrhea which may lead to dehydration and electrolyte imbalance [4–7].

5.2.2.6 Hematology

Related Problems

- In the cancer patient, **anemia** is most frequent.
- Hemorrhage, thrombosis and blastic blasts crisis are also found. The causes are diverse including chemotherapy, radiotherapy, bone marrow infiltration, sepsis, or coagulation disorders.
  - Hemorrhage is the second most common cause of death in patients with leukemia.
- Multiple drugs used in oncology patients such as asparaginase, actinomycin D, anthracyclines, antibiotics, or vincristine are frequently involved in coagulation disorders.

Anesthetics Measures

- In the preoperative blood tests, it is essential to have a complete blood count analysis and coagulation.
- Transfusion is necessary if the platelet count is below 50,000/μL. For prolonged surgical procedures, it would be desirable to be above 75,000/μL.
- White cells should be under 100,000/μL before surgery. Leukapheresis or exsanguination in younger children may be an option in emergency presentation of leukemia.
- Overall, it is extremely important before surgery to contact the blood bank and confirm the availability of appropriate blood products for the patient [2].

5.2.2.7 Infection

Anesthetics Measures

- Antibiotic prophylaxis must be performed in all surgical procedures following the guidelines of the infectious disease department at each institution according to the local epidemiology.
- Tetanus immunization is recommended, but not mandatory, before entering the operating room [8, 9].

5.2.2.8 Fasting

Anesthetics Measures

Table 5.2 Recommended fasting times [10]

Recommendation	Fasting times
Formula milk, baby food, and solid food	Up to 6 h before surgery or anesthesia
Breast milk only	Up to 4 h before surgery or anesthesia
Small amounts of water Quantity 3 mL/kg. Maximum 200 mL	Up to 1 h before surgery or anesthesia

See Table 5.2.

5.3 Anesthetic Management

1. Before entering the operating room

   Direct contact is made between the anesthesiologist, the family, and the patient. At this time it is necessary to confirm allergies, fasting, area of intervention, and relevant points of the patient's history and resolve any further doubts that the family or the child may have.
2. Induction

   For anesthetic induction it is highly recommended that parents be present until the child falls asleep. Cancer patients will undergo multiple anesthesias, and it is desirable to mitigate their psychological suffering as much as possible.
3. Maintenance

   Maintenance phase depends on whether it is a long surgery or a short anesthesia for a diagnostic or therapeutic test. However, some studies have suggested that propofol has a potential benefit as an anesthetic agent in patients with cancer promoting natural killer cell cytotoxicity, reduces tumor cell motility, and inhibits cyclooxygenase [11].

   Patient's temperature maintenance is extremely important. Hypothermia reduces in 5% the general metabolism. There is a reversible platelet dysfunction, due to thromboxane A2 alteration. It also increases the risk of surgical wound infection. At the cardiovascular level, it decreases the heart rate and increases oxygen consumption [12].
4. Waking up

   For short surgeries with little blood loss, it is better to awake the patient. On the other hand, in any of the following, patients should be remained intubated for several hours: patients under 3 years of age, who have undergone long surgeries, have significant blood loss, have been polytransfused, who have hypothermia, or who have poor pain control. In complex and aggressive surgeries, it is advisable to perform the postoperative period in critical care units.
5. Pain

   Perioperative pain can be approached in several ways. Peripheral or central blocks are an excellent option, but they cannot always be carried out either because of the location of the tumor or because of the large doses of anesthetics needed that could be toxic. A good alternative is the use of intravenous opioids. Patient-controlled analgesia (PCA) with morphine pumps and nurse-controlled analgesia (NCA) for younger children are commonly used with excellent results.

5.4 Tips and Tricks

5.4.1 Anesthesia for Central Line Placement

This is probably the most common procedure in surgical oncology.

Ultrasound-guided Seldinger technique is the most common and recommended approach when placing a central line. In the pediatric population, this procedure is usually performed under general anesthesia.

Besides ultrasound, intraoperative X-ray and cardiopulmonary monitorization are mandatory during central venous catheter (CVC) placement in order to avoid or promptly detect any possible complications.

5.4.2 Anesthesia for Neuroblastoma

Neuroblastoma (NB) is the most common extracranial solid tumor in childhood. Neuroblastoma surgery is probably the most demanding surgery in pediatric surgical oncology. Its location is usually intra-abdominal, although it can originate anywhere along the sympathetic chain.

Surgical Approaches and Anesthesia Considerations:

1. Cervical Neuroblastoma

   Primary cervical neuroblastoma represents between 3% and 5% of all locations, and additional cases can be the result of metastatic disease.

   Airway compression is uncommon and rarely described in cervical NB major case series. Depending on the tumor extension, an ultrasound-guided cervical block can be performed, which usually allows both deep and superficial anesthesia, granting good postoperative pain control in association with oral and intravenous analgesia [13].

2. Cervicothoracic Neuroblastoma

   Primary cervicothoracic NB usually arises from the stellate ganglion and progress extending in both directions, upward to the skull basis and downward to the posterior mediastinum.

   The first choice in cervicothoracic NB is general anesthesia associated with the insertion of an epidural catheter at the level of the thoracic spine, aiming to achieve analgesia both on the incision and on the site of chest tube insertion [13].

3. Thoracic Neuroblastoma

   Primary thoracic neuroblastoma represents approximately 14% of possible locations. The most common surgical approach is posterolateral thoracotomy, which provides good exposure and control of the mediastinum and allows a safe tumor resection. Video-assisted thoracoscopic surgery is a valuable approach for smaller lesions and allows the patient to benefit from minimal incisions and a lower rate of postoperative pain. Directly associated to a minimally invasive approach is one-lung ventilation (OLV).

   When thoracotomy is performed, anesthesia commonly involves general anesthetic drugs associated with the placement of an epidural catheter, as for the cervicothoracic tumors. General anesthesia associated with locoregional blockade is generally performed during thoracoscopic procedures.

4. Abdominal and Pelvic Neuroblastoma

   The presence of an abdominal mass increases intra-abdominal pressure (IAP). This increases the risk of aspiration; therefore rapid sequence induction is recommendable.

   The retroperitoneum is the most common location of NB, with adrenal glands being involved in 35% of cases. Surgical approaches change significantly according to the disease stage. Large masses with an extensive vascular encasement or lymph node dissemination require an open approach, consisting mainly of two different techniques: transverse abdominal laparotomy and thoracoabdominal exploration.

   Abdominal open surgery usually requires general anesthesia associated with a lumbar epidural catheter for intraoperative and postoperative analgesia. Sometimes an ultrasound-guided locoregional blockade is a feasible and reliable option.

5.4.3 Anesthesia for Kidney Tumors

Anesthetic management in patients with WT can be especially challenging and usually begins preoperatively because more than 25% of these patients have **hypertension**. Presumed mechanisms for hypertension include elevated renin levels secondary to renal ischemia produced by mechanical compression of the renal artery, secretion of renin by the tumor itself, and a possible pressor substance produced by the tumor.

Surgeon's Checklist

1. The preoperative contact of the anesthesiologist with the patient and his pathology is very important.
2. The anesthesia of the cancer patient should always be considered more complex than that of the patient without comorbidities and be prepared accordingly.
3. The type of tumor, its anatomical location, and the treatments received influence the anesthetic process.
4. One of the most complex anesthetic procedures in pediatric oncological surgery is neuroblastoma surgery.
5. Anesthetic management in this type of procedure focuses on pain control and airway patency.

References

1. Kuttesch JF, Raney RB. Principles of chemotherapy for solid tumors. In: Andrassy RJ, editor. Pediatric surgical oncology. Philadelphia: WB Saunders Company; 1998. p. 71–87.
2. Nesbitt KK, Massengill JB, Porche VH. Anesthesia, sedation, and pain management. In: Andrassy RJ, editor. Pediatric surgical oncology. Philadelphia: WB Saunders Company; 1998. p. 35–69.
3. Balis FM, Holcenberg JS, Blaney SM. General principles of chemotherapy. In: Pizzo PA, Poplack DG, editors. Principles and practice of pediatric oncology. 4th ed. Philadelphia: Lippincott Williams & Wilkins; 2002. p. 237–308.
4. Andrassy RJ. General principles. In: Andrassy RJ, editor. Pediatric surgical oncology. Philadelphia: WB Saunders Company; 1998. p. 13–34.
5. Krane EJ, Domino KB. Anesthesia for neurosurgery. In: Motoyama EK, Davis PJ, editors. Smith's anesthesia for infants and children. 6th ed. St Louis: Mosby-Year Book; 1996. p. 541–70.
6. Haberkern CM. Neuroblastoma. In: Stheling L, editor. Common problems in pediatric anesthesia. 2th ed. St Louis: Mosby-Year Book; 1992. p. 177–82.
7. Bissonnette B, Sadeghi P. Anesthesia for neurosurgical procedures. In: Gregory GA, editor. Pediatric anesthesia. 4th ed. New York: Churchill Livingstone; 2002. p. 381–422.
8. Alexandes SW, Walsh TJ, Freifeld AG, Pizzo PA. Infectious complications in pediatric cancer patients. In: Pizzo PA, Poplack DG, editors. Principles and practice of pediatric oncology. 4th ed. Philadelphia: Lippincott Williams & Wilkins; 2002. p. 1239–83.
9. Han I, Viscoli C, Paesmans M, et al. A comparison of outcome from febrile neutropenic episodes in children compared with adults results from four EORTC studies. International Antimicrobial Therapy Cooperative Group (IATCG) of the European Organization.
10. Frykholm P, Disma N, Andersson H, Beck C, Bouvet L, Cercueil E, Elliott E, Hofmann J, Isserman R, Klaucane A, Kuhn F, de Queiroz Siqueira M, Rosen D, Rudolph D, Schmidt AR, Schmitz A, Stocki D, Sümpelmann R, Stricker PA, Thomas M, Veyckemans F, Afshari A. Preoperative fasting in children: A guideline from the European Society of Anaesthesiology and Intensive Care. Eur J Anaesthesiol. 2022;39(1):4–25. https://doi.org/10.1097/EJA.0000000000001599. PMID: 34857683.
11. Capote G. Why propofol in cancer patient? Rev Chil Anest. 2019;48:223–9.
12. Crisóstomo MM, Hernández AL, Ordoñez G, Riera C. Hypothermia and its effects during anesthesia in children. Rev Mexicana Pediatr. 2011;78(4):131–8.
13. Shamberger RC, Holzman RS, Griscom NT, Tarbell NJ, Weinstein HJ. CT quantitation of tracheal cross-sectional area as a guide to the surgical and anesthetic management of children with anterior mediastinal masses. J Pediatr Surg. 1991;26(2):138–42. https://doi.org/10.1016/0022-3468(91)90894-y. PMID: 2023069.

6 Biopsy Procedures and Practical Issues

Nelson Piché

For many families of children afflicted by cancer, the diagnostic biopsy will be their first experience with an invasive procedure. This important step in management must be carefully planned to minimize the discomfort to the patient and the risk of potential complications, including the need for repeat procedures, while ensuring appropriate tissue sampling for accurate diagnosis and risk level assignment. Pediatric surgeons coordinating this process must consider several factors such as the local expertise available, the suspected diagnosis, the tumor site and stage, and the overall general condition of the patient. While a biopsy procedure is most frequently performed for diagnostic purposes, all the following concepts also apply for assessment of potential metastatic disease, confirmation of recurrence, or evaluation of treatment response.

6.1 Is a Biopsy Indicated or Necessary?

The indication and value of a biopsy must be carefully determined for each patient. Pediatric surgeons should understand the overall management plan and the anticipated patient trajectory of care before proceeding.

N. Piché (✉)
Pediatric Surgery, CHU Ste-Justine, Université de Montréal, Montreal, QC, Canada
e-mail: nelson.piche.med@ssss.gouv.qc.ca

In general, if a tumor can be resected entirely with a margin of normal tissue without functional or cosmetic sequelae, then an excisional biopsy or upfront resection could be favored over an incisional or percutaneous biopsy. The incision should be positioned adequately (see below), and the specimen must be sent oriented with identification of any suspicious margins.

Most research protocols and treatment plans mandate diagnosis by tissue sampling. However, it is sometimes possible to establish a diagnosis and begin treatment without a biopsy. Examples include bilateral Wilms tumors, neuroblastoma patients with elevated homovanillic acid (HVA) and vanillylmandelic acid (VMA) and a positive Meta-Iodo-Benzyl-Guanidine (MIBG) study (intermediate risk neuroblastoma patients will require biopsy for molecular and other biological studies; see Chap. 11) or older patients with a typical sacrococcygeal tumor on imaging and elevated serum alpha-fetoprotein (AFP). While these situations are infrequent, pediatric surgeons should consider this possibility, especially for patients with fragile functional status or when biopsy could lead to complications and treatment delays. Patients managed without initial biopsy require close imaging surveillance and prompt biopsy in case of inadequate response to therapy.

Involvement of parents in the decision process has tremendous value and has proven to be beneficial in many aspects of pediatric care [1].

L. Krauel (ed.), *Survival Handbook in Pediatric Surgical Oncology*,
https://doi.org/10.1007/978-3-031-65890-7_6

Pediatric surgeons must include parents and families in the preparation for biopsy.

6.2 Patient and Tumor Characteristics

The work-up of a pediatric patient presenting with a tumor should include oncologic staging and functional status of the child. In preparation for biopsy, the initial assessment should include complete blood work with coagulation, cardiopulmonary and airway functions, and nutritional status.

The presumed histologic diagnosis will influence the decision process for biopsy. For several pediatric malignant tumors, a biopsy will upstage the tumor and consequently must be avoided if a complete upfront resection can be achieved safely (e.g., Wilms tumor, germ cell tumor, and hepatoblastoma). Conversely, the optimal strategy sometimes involves a diagnostic incisional or percutaneous biopsy, potentially followed by neoadjuvant chemotherapy. Notable examples for this situation are L2 neuroblastomas [2], suspected Ewing's sarcomas of the chest wall which require radiation therapy if the resection margin is positive [3], and large/bulky malignant germ cell tumors of the mediastinum [4] and retroperitoneum [5].

While an exhaustive review for each tumor type is beyond the scope of this chapter, Table 6.1

Table 6.1 Usual role of diagnostic biopsy for selected pediatric solid malignancies. Please refer to the specific chapters for details regarding each tumor type

Presumed diagnosis	Usual role of biopsy
Neuroblastoma	• Biopsy indicated for L2 tumors, most cases of metastatic disease and for Ms disease • Requires 1–2 cm^3 of tissue or 20+ cores using 14-gauge core needle • L1 tumors usually resected upfront
Kidney tumor	• Biopsy is contraindicated in most cases • Children oncology group (COG): most stages I to IV will undergo upfront resection Biopsy only if tumors deemed unresectable by exploration, tumor thrombus extending to retro-hepatic cava, and pulmonary compromise from bulky primary or pulmonary metastasis • International society of paediatric oncology (SIOP): neoadjuvant chemotherapy for tumors with typical clinical features. Biopsy if atypical presentation, no response or progression during neoadjuvant chemotherapy • Treatment for Stage V (bilateral) and tumor in a solitary kidney are usually initiated without biopsy
Liver tumor	• Biopsy indicated for PRETEXT II with less than 1-cm margin, PRETEXT III and IV tumors • PRETEXT I and PRETEXT II with more than 1-cm margin usually resected upfront • Requires 1 cm^3 of tissue or >10 cores using 16-gauge core needle and should include normal liver tissue
Rhabdomyosarcoma	• Biopsy indicated if resection would cause unacceptable functional or cosmetic morbidity • Sample clinically positive nodes • *Testicular*: biopsy not indicated in most cases and upfront excision preferred if possible
Germ cells tumours (GCT)	• *Mediastinum and retroperitoneal*: initial biopsy and delayed resection for bulky/invasive tumors • *Testicular*: biopsy not indicated in most cases and upfront excision preferred if possible. Transscrotal approach and biopsy will upstage • *Ovarian*: Biopsy not indicated in most cases. Usually resectable upfront. Incomplete peritoneal staging or biopsy will cause upstage • *Sacrococcygeal teratoma (SCT)*: usually resected upfront at birth. Late presentation associated with large unresectable lesion; biopsy followed by neoadjuvant chemotherapy
Sarcomas	• Always orient specimen and identify margins • *Chest wall*: usual initial biopsy followed by neoadjuvant chemotherapy

summarizes the role of biopsy for the diagnosis of selected pediatric cancers. Please refer to the respective chapters of this textbook for more details.

When a diagnostic biopsy is indicated, it is usually preferable to sample the primary tumor. However, if distant disease (nodal or metastatic) can be biopsied with significantly less morbidity, then it should be considered. An important example for this concept is the patient that presents with airway compromise from an anterior mediastinal tumor: sampling pleural effusion or nodal disease using local anesthesia may prove diagnostic while being safer [6].

If metabolic imaging has been performed, areas of high activity should be preferentially targeted, especially in large and heterogeneous lesions.

6.3 Choice of Approach

Traditionally, surgeons provided a tumor specimen for pathologic analysis with an incisional or excisional biopsy using an open or minimally invasive approach. However, the image-guided percutaneous approach has been used with increased frequency in recent years with satisfactory results for several types of tumors [7] including neuroblastoma [8, 9], hepatoblastoma [10], and soft-tissue sarcoma [11]. Both approaches have distinctive advantages and drawbacks that must be considered when planning a biopsy procedure.

Whether open or percutaneous, the biopsy incision or needle tract must be excised for most tumors and for all sarcomas. Consequently, the site and orientation of the biopsy must be planned with the final resection in mind. Furthermore, tumor heterogeneity and potential spillage must also be carefully considered.

When the technical installations and medical skills are available locally to perform a percutaneous biopsy, several potential advantages have been reported in the literature for this approach, including decreased transfusion rate, decreased post-procedural pain, a quicker return of function, and improved cost-effectiveness. The procedure can sometimes be performed using sedation, or even local anesthesia in selected cases, rather than general anesthesia, precluding the need for orotracheal intubation. However, the position of the tumor may not provide a safe window for percutaneous biopsy, and if the number of needle core samples obtained is not sufficient, the amount of tissue provided for analysis may be inadequate.

Most centers performing image-guided percutaneous biopsies use a coaxial technique with 14- or 16-gauge needles and ultrasound or computed tomography (CT) guidance. The optimal number of core needle samples obtained is currently being investigated and varies by tumor type. Discussion with pathology, oncology, and molecular biology teams prior to the procedure is important in this regard. Tumors that are heterogeneous on imaging or that may require elaborate work-up like molecular sequencing (e.g., neuroblastoma) should lead to obtention of a greater number of core needle samples. Hemostatic agents like gelatin or collagen sponges are sometimes embolized in the biopsy tract as the needle is withdrawn [12] to minimize bleeding risk.

When percutaneous biopsy is not available or deemed inappropriate because of tumor or patient characteristics, the surgical biopsy can be performed using open or minimally invasive techniques.

For bone and soft-tissue tumor biopsy, trunk incisions are generally oriented transversely and limb incisions longitudinally (parallel to the axis of the limb). For large tumors that may eventually require reconstruction, early involvement of onco-plastic colleagues should be considered. Hepatic biopsies should only pass through liver segments that will be excised at the time of final resection and be planned as to carefully avoid peritoneal spillage. In the infrequent instance that a renal biopsy is required, spillage must be avoided, and if a percutaneous approach is used, a tract that avoids peritoneal seeding should be used if possible. Transscrotal biopsies should be avoided: testicular lesions are managed by an inguinal approach. Likewise, abdominal and thoracic incisions should be planned with the goal of being resected at the time of final tumor resection.

When a tumor is heterogeneous, sampling of different areas of the primary tumor should be considered. And as mentioned previously, areas of high metabolic activity, as demonstrated on positron emission tomography (PET) scanning when available, should be targeted if possible. Tumors may displace adjacent organs, and the normal anatomical relationships between structures may be lost, especially in smaller children. Careful avoidance of vital structures must be exercised, and meticulous revision of preprocedural imaging is of utmost importance. Once the biopsy site is identified and isolated from surrounding structures, the capsule of the tumor is opened, and the specimen is acquired using the knife blade, scissors, or a rongeur. Cautery and other heat sources are avoided to prevent specimen degradation. After obtaining sufficient tissue (1–3 cm^3 per site), the biopsy cavity is filled with hemostatic agent (e.g., thrombin-infused gelfoam), and pressure is applied until adequate hemostasis is obtained. Excessive use of cautery to attain hemostasis can lead to heat injury to adjacent organs. If a minimally invasive approach is used, the specimen should be retrieved in a bag to decrease the potential risk of spillage and port site recurrence.

Communication with the attending pathologist *prior* to the biopsy procedure is important to ensure that the specimen will be handled adequately. The biopsy tissue should be sent fresh, never in formalin, immediately after its procurement. Some teams have a pediatric pathologist present in the procedure room at the time of biopsy to assess and improve the adequacy of tissue sampling [9].

Another important aspect in the planification of a diagnostic biopsy is the consideration for central venous access placement and bone marrow aspirates/biopsy. When these interventions are clinically indicated, efforts should be made to perform them during the same procedure thus avoiding repeat potential anesthetic risks. Furthermore, for suspected bone and soft-tissue sarcoma, regional lymph nodes that are clinically or radiologically positive should be sampled for adequate staging.

Complication from the biopsy procedure can cause delay in systemic therapy initiation. The most frequently reported complications include infection and bleeding. As mentioned previously, the normal anatomical relationship between organs can be altered by bulky tumors, and this should be taken into consideration to avoid iatrogenic injury. Blood type and blood products should be readily available for all intracavitary procedures and for biopsies performed near significant blood vessels. Patients with heavy tumor burden are considered immunocompromised, and antibioprophylaxis should be administered at anesthesia induction.

In conclusion, the objective of a biopsy procedure is to secure a definitive diagnosis promptly and safely. Several factors related to the tumor and the patient must be considered in order to choose the optimal approach for each patient, and thus pediatric surgeons are best suited to lead the process of biopsy planning.

Surgeon's Checklist

1. Coordinate procedure planification with oncology, pathology, and interventional radiology to determine the amount of tissue needed and the optimal approach for the biopsy.
2. Involve family in the decision process, and document consent according to local practices.
3. Obtain preoperative anesthesia consultation, especially for mediastinal tumors and for patients with low functional reserve.
4. Consider all disease sites: diagnosis can be established from primary, nodal, or distant disease and sometimes from effusions.
5. Plan biopsy site and skin incision carefully. Biopsy incision and track should be selected with definitive resection in mind. Biopsy tract will need to be resected in most patients and for all sarcomas.
6. Consider that some lesions may not need biopsy to initiate therapy (e.g., bilateral Wilms, high-risk neuroblastoma with positive MIBG and urinary catecholamines, etc.).
7. Consider upfront resection rather than biopsy (e.g., L1 NB, Wilms tumors, PRETEXT I and some PRETEXT II liver tumors, etc.).
8. Consider need for other invasive procedures (e.g., tunneled central venous access, bone marrow aspirate/biopsy) to avoid unnecessary repeat anesthesia.
9. Administer antibioprophylaxis at induction of anesthesia.

References

1. Loeff DS, Shakhsheer BA. The ethics of informed consent and shared decision-making in pediatric surgery. Semin Pediatr Surg. 2021;30(5):151101.
2. Newman EA, Abdessalam S, Aldrink JH, Austin M, Heaton TE, Bruny J, et al. Update on neuroblastoma. J Pediatr Surg. 2019;54(3):383–9.
3. Shamberger RC, LaQuaglia MP, Gebhardt MC, Neff JR, Tarbell NJ, Marcus KC, et al. Ewing sarcoma/primitive neuroectodermal tumor of the chest wall: impact of initial versus delayed resection on tumor margins, survival, and use of radiation therapy. Ann Surg. 2003;238(4):563–7; discussion 567–8.
4. Schneider DT, Calaminus G, Reinhard H, Gutjahr P, Kremens B, Harms D, et al. Primary mediastinal germ cell tumors in children and adolescents: results of the German cooperative protocols MAKEI 83/86, 89, and 96. J Clin Oncol. 2000;18(4):832–9.
5. Billmire D, Vinocur C, Rescorla F, Colombani P, Cushing B, Hawkins E, et al. Malignant retroperitoneal and abdominal germ cell tumors: an intergroup study. J Pediatr Surg. 2003;38(3):315–8; discussion 318.
6. Perger L, Lee EY, Shamberger RC. Management of children and adolescents with a critical airway due to compression by an anterior mediastinal mass. J Pediatr Surg. 2008;43(11):1990–7.
7. Serati L, Morosi C, Barretta F, Collini P, Calareso G, Chiaravalli S, et al. Diagnostic yield and accuracy of image-guided percutaneous core needle biopsy of paediatric solid tumours: an experience from Italy. Pediatr Hematol Oncol J. 2021;6(1):12–7.
8. Campagna G, Rosenfeld E, Foster J, Vasudevan S, Nuchtern J, Kim E, et al. Evolving biopsy techniques for the diagnosis of neuroblastoma in children. J Pediatr Surg. 2018;53(11):2235–9.
9. Overman RE, Kartal TT, Cunningham AJ, Fialkowski EA, Naik-Mathuria BJ, Vasudevan SA, et al. Optimization of percutaneous biopsy for diagnosis and pretreatment risk assessment of neuroblastoma. Pediatr Blood Cancer. 2020;67(5):e28153.
10. Weldon CB, Madenci AL, Tiao GM, Dunn SP, Langham MR, McGahren ED, et al. Evaluation of the diagnostic biopsy approach for children with hepatoblastoma: a report from the Children's Oncology Group AHEP 0731 Liver Tumor Committee. J Pediatr Surg. 2020;55(4):655–9.
11. Cooke-Barber J, Brungardt JG, Sorger M, Pressey JG, Turpin B, Nagarajan R, et al. Pediatric and young adult image-guided percutaneous bone biopsy-a new standard of care? Ann Surg Oncol. 2023;30(6):3658–65.
12. Metz T, Heider A, Vellody R, Jarboe MD, Gemmete JJ, Grove JJ, et al. Image-guided percutaneous core needle biopsy of soft-tissue masses in the pediatric population. Pediatr Radiol. 2016;46(8):1173–8.

Vascular Access in Pediatric Oncology

7

Marta Pilar Martin Giménez and Albert Pasten

7.1 Introduction

Central venous access device (CVAD) placement is one of the most common procedures in pediatric surgical oncology. In some centers this procedure is carried out by the anesthesiologist or interventional radiology. However, it is frequent for the placement of fully or partially implantable devices, such as port-a-caths and apheresis catheters, to be performed by pediatric surgeons. We will describe the different types of available devices, insertion techniques, anatomical locations, and potential complications.

7.2 Types of Central Venous Catheters

Central venous access devices (CVADs) are generally classified based on the duration of the catheter use; thus we will find short-term, mid-term, and long-term devices. Also related to dwell time, we will find if the catheter is implanted or not and to what extent (tunneled or totally implanted) (Table 7.1). Another aspect to take in consideration is the diameter of the catheter, as this will be important to calculate maximum flow rate.

Non-tunneled catheters: These catheters are most commonly used for temporary venous access. Usually are placed percutaneously with the catheter exiting the skin next to the venous cannulation site (jugular, subclavian, femoral).

Peripherally inserted central catheters (PICCs) are another type of non-tunneled catheters. These devices are popular due to the relative ease of insertion into the peripheral veins of the upper extremity (brachial vein, basilic vein), a lower risk of insertion-related complications, and improved patient tolerance.

Tunneled catheters: Tunneled central venous catheters traverse a subcutaneous tunnel between

Table 7.1 Types of central devices

Catheter type	Entry site	Duration of use
Non tunneled	Internal jugular vein, subclavian, femoral (central veins)	Days to weeks
PICCs	Basilic or cephalic vein. Long saphenous vein. Tip of the catheter in the central vein	Weeks to months
Tunneled	Subcutaneous tunnel with cuffed catheter into central vein	Months to years
Totally implanted	Port positioned usually on chest wall with subcutaneous tunneled portion to central vein	Months to years

M. P. M. Giménez (✉) · A. Pasten
Pediatric Surgical Oncology, Pediatric Surgery Department, Pediatric Cancer Center Barcelona (PCCB), SJD Barcelona Children's Hospital, Universitat de Barcelona, Barcelona, Spain
e-mail: martapilar.martin@sjd.es; albert.pasten@sjd.es

L. Krauel (ed.), *Survival Handbook in Pediatric Surgical Oncology*,
https://doi.org/10.1007/978-3-031-65890-7_7

the catheterized vein and the skin exit site. Generally these catheters have a cuff (Velour®, Dacron®) that is positioned in the subcutaneous tissue adjacent to the exit site to anchor the catheter and create a fibrous barrier to skin pathogens. In general, rates of infection associated with tunneled catheters are lower compared with non-tunneled central venous catheters.

Totally implanted (ports): They are placed entirely under the skin tissue (no skin exit site). The catheter of these devices passes from the cannulated vein beneath the skin and is attached to a subcutaneous infusion port that is placed into a subcutaneous pocket.

These are meant to be permanent, with removal reserved when complications occur, the device is no longer needed (completion of treatment), or patient comfort. Subcutaneous ports have the advantage of concealment from view and protection from the overlying skin, making this option more cosmetically appealing and compatible with activities such as bathing or swimming.

Tunneled cuffed catheters and implanted ports are generally associated with lower rates of catheter-related bloodstream infection compared with non-implanted catheters.

7.3 Insertion Techniques

Centrally inserted catheters are primarily placed via the internal jugular vein (IJV), subclavian vein, or femoral vein and advanced until the terminal lumen resides within the inferior vena cava, superior vena cava, or right atrium. Alternative insertion sites include the external jugular vein and cephalic vein; these usually are cannulated by using a cutdown technique.

We are going to focus on the ultrasound (US)-guided Seldinger technique [1]. This procedure has remained rather unchanged since its description in the 1960s, aside from the use of US guidance [2], which has become the standard of care for central venous catheters (CVCs) placed in the internal jugular vein, owing to associated decreases in complications and an increase in first attempt success.

Based on randomized trials and observational studies demonstrating lower complication rates and other benefits, we suggest placement of an implantable, subcutaneous port device, rather than a tunneled catheter (i.e., Hickman) or PICC. Because port placement requires an interventional or surgical procedure, immediate availability may be limited. PICC placement (fewest number of lumens) is a reasonable option when port placement is not immediately feasible (or contraindicated) and can serve as a short-term bridge to port placement especially if long-term, intermittent, or cyclical therapy is planned.

For implantable port access for cancer therapy, a trial comparing the internal jugular with subclavian site also found no significant difference in infection rates [3].

7.4 Percutaneous Techniques (IJV)

1. General anesthesia and oral intubation.
2. Supine position and head turned away from the insertion site. Trendelenburg position. The choice of the vein depends on the surgeon's preference, patient anatomy, and history of site use.
3. Surgical draping for the neck and upper chest using chlorhexidine solution. The surgeon will be positioned behind the patient's head or next to the puncture site.
4. Under ultrasound guidance, identify the vein (compressible) (Fig. 7.1). Position the probe covered with a sterile bag containing gel, at the apex of the sternomastoid triangle at the base of the neck. Usually in children we use the short-axis view.
5. With the needle given in the catheter kit of choice or a micropuncture access set, attached to a 10 cc syringe with 2–3 cc of saline, puncture the vessel at a 45°–90° angle, and advance the hand through the skin, holding negative pressure on the syringe until a flash of dark venous blood appears. Be sure to maintain dynamic visualization of the needle tip as it enters the vessel (Fig. 7.2).

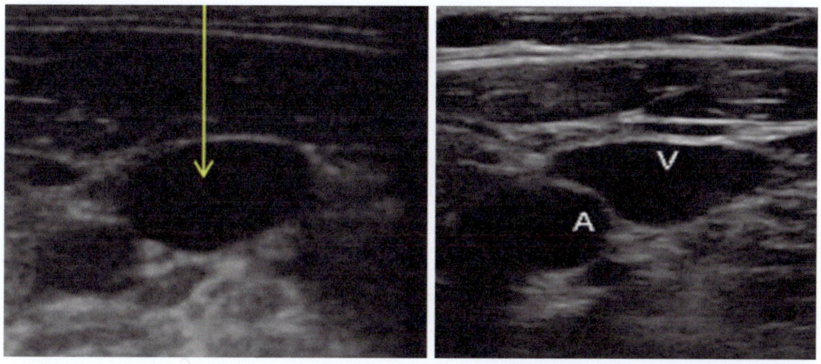

Fig. 7.1 Ultrasonographic landmarks for finding internal jugular vein

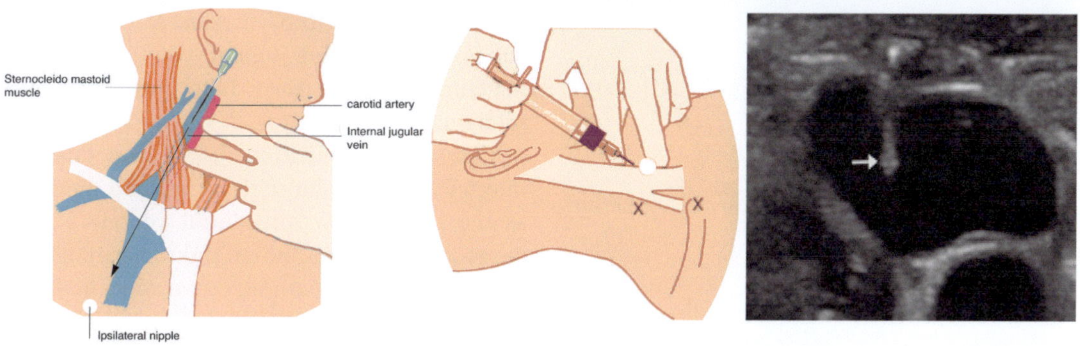

Fig. 7.2 Depiction of angle and ultrasonographic vision of the needle

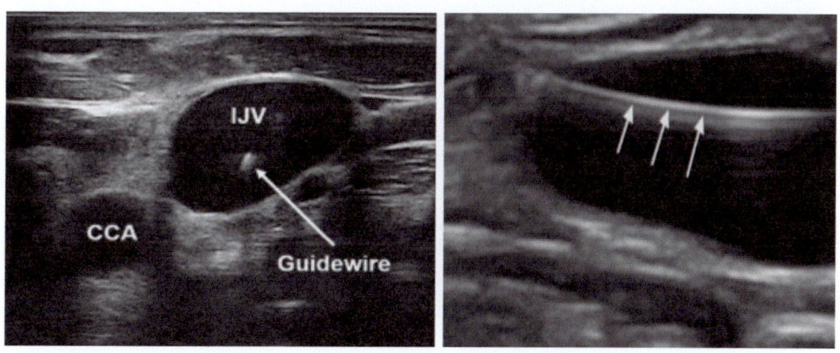

Fig. 7.3 Ultrasonographic vision of the guidewire in transverse and longitudinal views

6. Introduce the guidewire through the needle following Seldinger technique principles (Fig. 7.3). It is importat to constantly check drooling of blood once the syringe is disconnected from the needle previous to continue with the next step.
7. Use fluoroscopy to confirm the position of the wire and the extent of its distal end (Fig. 7.4). Pass the introducer sheath over the wire, then remove wire, and introduce the catheter through the sheath.
8. Check out catheter positioning with fluoroscopy leaving the tip of the catheter close to the entrance of the right atrium. Use the right main bronchus as anatomical landmark. Use a 10 cc syringe filled with 3–4 cc of saline connected to the catheter to verify proper functioning.

Once the vascular time is done, depending on what kind of device is being used:

1. Port-a-cath: Creation of subcutaneous pocket. Usually one finger breadth below the clavicle (middle third). Open by planes until the pectoral fascia. Tunnel the catheter through the pectoral incision to the neck or from the neck to the port location. Connect all device components. The portal is then fixed with two absorbable sutures to the fascia.
2. Tunneled catheter: Mark the catheter exit site, and then incised with a scalpel. Using a tunneler with a tapered tip at one end and the catheter attached at the other end, the catheter is tunneled along the subcutaneous tissue from the chest wall over the clavicle and toward the neck.

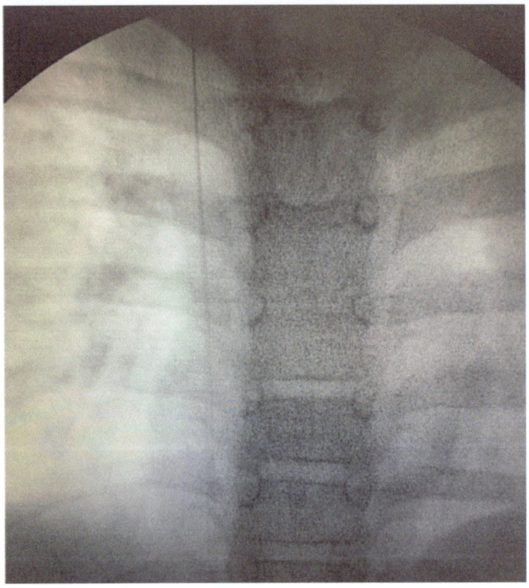

Fig. 7.4 Fluoroscopic vision of the guidewire in right atrial position

Many centers use the subclavian vein for central access (Fig. 7.5). Seldinger technique using anatomical references is well described and has a high rate of success in experienced hands. The internal jugular vein also can be punctured with the help of anatomic references.

Our recommendation is to puncture the internal jugular vein with ultrasound guidance as the first option for central venous access, because it's a safe and straightforward procedure, with a little learning curve and a high rate of success.

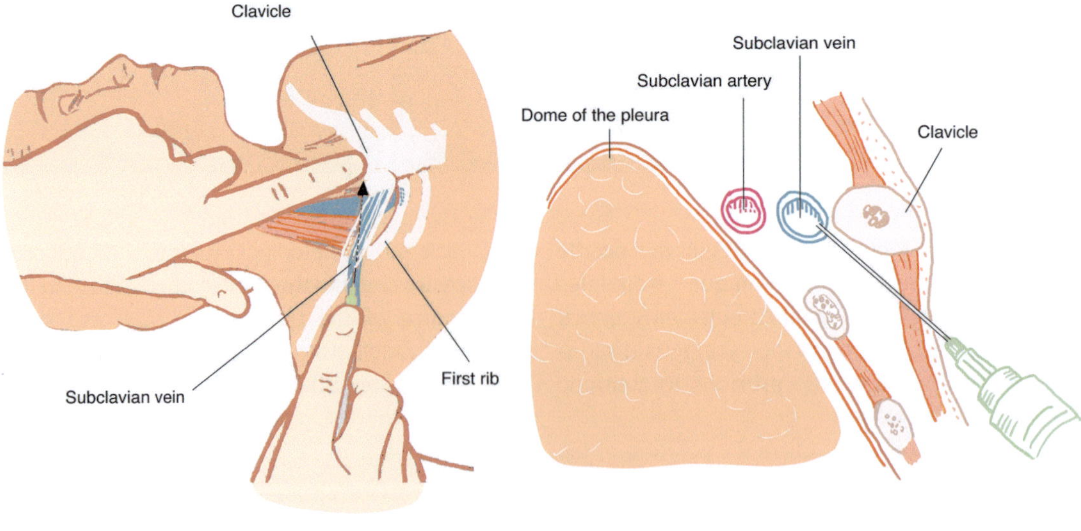

Fig. 7.5 Schematic depiction of Seldinger technique for subclavian vein access

7.5 Cutdown Techniques

Limited experience or access to an ultrasound can be challenging sometimes, so venous cutdown is a safe option. A careful surgical approach will warrant a phlebotomy without damage; therefore anatomic knowledge and tips for vein identification are very important.

The most used veins for cutdown are the following:

- External jugular vein: It can be found in the lateral aspect of the neck, running from lateral to medial from mandibular angle to middle third of clavicle, superficial to sternocleidomastoid muscle. If it's not visible, the patient can be positioned in Trendelenburg position and/or press the right hypochondrium to promote blood reflux from the liver.
- Cephalic vein: It can be found in the deltopectoral groove, medial to the humeral head and inferior to the clavicle. Between the fibers of pectoralis major and deltoid muscles, the avascular groove is dissected to expose cephalic vein.
- Internal jugular vein: It can be found deep to sternocleidomastoid muscle, anterolateral to common carotid artery. After exposing the vein, it is useful to get vascular control by vessel loops and do a purse-string suture with polypropylene. Inside this, a phlebotomy is performed, the catheter is introduced, and then the purse string can be closed.

Table 7.2 summarizes the most common veins used for vascular access and its advantages and disadvantages.

Table 7.2 Specific anatomic sites and access approaches with their inherent advantages and disadvantages

Approach	Advantages	Disadvantages
External jugular	Superficial vessel that is often visible Coagulopathy not prohibitive Minimal risk of pneumothorax Head-of-table access Prominent in older adult patients Rapid venous access	Poor landmarks in patients with obesity High rate of malposition Catheter may be difficult to thread
Internal jugular	Minimal risk of pneumothorax (especially with US guidance) Head-of-table access Procedure-related bleeding amenable to direct pressure Lower failure rate with novice operator Excellent target using US guidance	Risk of carotid artery puncture Uncomfortable (if external) Thoracic duct injury possible on left Poor landmarks in patients with obesity/ edematous patients Potential access and maintenance issues with concomitant tracheostomy Vein prone to collapse with hypovolemia
Subclavian	Easier to maintain dressings More comfortable for patient Better landmarks in patients with obesity Accessible when airway control is being established Associated with lower incidence of catheter-related infection[a] [1]	Increased risk of pneumothorax Procedure-related bleeding less amenable to direct pressure Decreased success rate with inexperience Longer path from skin to vessel Catheter malposition more common (especially right superior vena cava (SVC) Risk for stenosis/occlusion, which impacts future hemodialysis arteriovenous access
Femoral	Rapid access with high success rate Does not interfere with intubation No risk of pneumothorax Trendelenburg position not necessary during insertion	Prevents patient mobilization Difficult to keep site sterile Difficult for PA catheter insertion Increased risk of iliofemoral thrombosis

7.6 Absolute Contraindications

Severe, uncorrectable coagulopathies, uncontrolled sepsis, and/or bacteremia are absolute contraindications to the placement of all tunneled CVCs. In these patients, a temporary, non-tunneled catheter should be placed until the coagulopathy can be corrected or the infection clears.

Recommended platelet counts:
- Internal jugular vein puncture >40,000/mm^3
- Subclavian vein puncture >80,000/mm^3
- Cutdown techniques >40,000/mm^3

7.7 Complications

Numerous potential complications can occur during the placement of a central venous catheter but also due to the indwelling equipment.

Procedural complications:
- Arrhythmias—typically ventricular or bundle branch blocks due to guidewire irritation of the atria or ventricles
- Arterial puncture
- Pulmonary puncture with or without pneumothorax
- Bleeding—hematoma formation, which can obstruct the airway
- Tracheal injury
- Air emboli during venipuncture or removal of the catheter

Post-procedural complications:
- Catheter-related bloodstream infections—bacterial or fungal
- Central vein stenosis
- Thrombosis
- Delayed bleeding with multiple attempts in a coagulopathic patient [4]

Intraoperative bleeding, hemo/pneumothorax, and arterial puncture are the most important. These three incidents can occur in subclavian puncture, and its management could become hard due to the difficult approach to this vein. A pleural drain will be sufficient for a pneumothorax, but for massive bleeding and hemothorax, a thoracotomy, sternotomy or trap-door (see Chap. 9) approach could be necessary for hemostasia. Arterial puncture can be suspected by high flux of blood in the puncture moment. If it occurs in the internal jugular vein, pressure can be applied for hemostasis.

Acute complications appearing after the procedure are infection, dysfunction, and displacement. The former one is infrequent but if fever and/or inflammatory changes in the skin overlying reservoir or catheter appear, at the third to fifth day postoperative, catheter infection should be suspected. Difficult to reflux or infuse is a sign of dysfunction and can reflect a disconnection from the reservoir or an incorrect placement of the tip that could generate a "wall effect" in the vein.

Chronic complications are infections, dysfunction, and accidental removal. The latter could occur in external catheters, tunneled or not, and unfortunately are not infrequent in children. Nurse care and good attachments are important for central line care. Infection is a permanent fear in immunosuppressed patients, and meticulous manipulation of central lines, with sterile technique and by experienced professionals, is crucial. Table 7.3 summarizes the diagnosis criteria for catheter-related infections (CRIs) and their management. Dysfunction could be due to line fracture, disconnection from reservoir, obstruction in the tip, or reservoir damage. Any of these warrants a surgical revision for placement of or removal.

Table 7.3 Summary recommendations for diagnostic procedures of catheter-related infections

Based on catheter withdrawal	Positive	Negative
When there is suspicion of CRI, at least two pairs of blood cultures using aseptic technique must be obtained	Start antimicrobial treatment Remove if infected by difficult-to-eradicate microorganisms	Keep device
When there are local signs of infection, a smear of the exudate should be sent for Gram staining and culture	Start antimicrobial treatment based on culture	Remove if the infection extend to the subcutaneous tunnel
Whenever possible to remove the catheter, culture of the tip. The port must be sent in addition to the catheter tip for culture in case of a totally implanted device	Change antimicrobial treatment based on culture	Wrong technique during sample taking Successful antimicrobial treatment

Surgeon's Checklist

1. Confirm with the treating team the type of catheter and diameter that are needed.
2. Be aware of the presence of other tunneled catheters such as ventriculoperitoneal shunts.
3. Verify the "vein status" of the patient before scheduling the procedure: if he/she has previously used a central line and if there is a history of thrombosis. Request a Doppler ultrasound if any of these antecedents are positive.
4. Check you have all the supplies necessary to perform the procedure, whether it will be done by ultrasound-guided puncture or by cutdown.
5. Choose a catheter caliber that will be sufficient to warrant a good function.
6. Reassure your guide or catheter is inside the vein before moving forward, especially when performing Seldinger technique.
7. Check you have good catheter flow.
8. Perform X-ray control. If you have used a roll underneath the shoulders, make sure it is out especially in small children as the tip of your catheter can slide in.
9. Check for possible complications.
10. Once the device is completely implanted/tunneled, check its function. Blood reflux and infusion should be smooth.
11. Cover the device under sterile conditions before the patient leaves the operating room. Mark the date on a visible position in order to keep track of possible changes of dressing.

References

1. Seldinger SI. Catheter replacement of the needle in percutaneous arteriography; a new technique. Acta Radiol. 1953;39(5):368–76.
2. Seldinger SI. Catheter replacement of the needle in percutaneous arteriography. A new technique. Acta Radiol Suppl (Stockholm). 2008;434:47–52. https://doi.org/10.1080/02841850802133386.
3. Biffi R, et al. Best choice of central venous insertion site for the prevention of catheter-related complications in adult patients who need cancer therapy: a randomized trial. Oncologia. 2009;20(5):935–40. https://doi.org/10.1093/annonc/mdn701.
4. van de Weerdt EK, Biemond BJ, Baake B, Vermin B, Binnekade JM, van Lienden KP, Vlaar APJ. Central venous catheter placement in coagulopathic patients: risk factors and incidence of bleeding complications. Transfusion. 2017;57(10):2512–25. https://doi.org/10.1111/trf.14248.

Management of Enlarged Lymph Nodes

8

Albert Pasten and Lucas Krauel

8.1 Introduction

Lymphadenopathy is a very common condition affecting children. The causes are very broad, mostly benign, and many times have an indolent course, remitting spontaneously without any intervention. However, an enlarged lymph node could be a sign of cancer or other severe conditions, and the surgeon should have guidelines for taking decisions and help to obtain a diagnosis [1].

The body has about 600 lymph nodes, and their function is to drain the extracellular fluid of antigens. When it's possible to palpate a normal lymph node, it's soft, mobile, and compressible. The location of each one defines the drainage region and could orientate about the origin of the pathology that causes an enlargement (Table 8.1) [1, 2].

Lymphadenopathy is defined as a lymph node with 1 cm or more of diameter (1.5 cm in the

Table 8.1 Lymph node location, its drainage zones, and differential diagnosis [1, 2]

Location	Drainage zone	Benign differential	Malignant differential
Cervical	Head and neck	Skin and odontogenic infections, viral, TB	Lymphoma, skin malignancies
Supraclavicular	Thorax (right), abdomen (left)	TB, fungal, viral	Thorax or abdomen malignancy
Infraclavicular	Mediastinum, thorax	TB, fungal, viral	Lymphoma
Axillary	Arm, breast, thorax, neck	Skin infection, Bartonella, trauma	Lymphoma, leukemia, melanoma, STS
Inguinal	Leg, abdominal wall, external genitalia	Skin infection, STI	Lymphoma, skin cancer, STS

TB tuberculosis, *STS* soft tissue sarcoma, *STI* sexually transmitted infection

A. Pasten (✉) · L. Krauel
Pediatric Surgical Oncology, Pediatric Surgery Department, Pediatric Cancer Center Barcelona (PCCB), SJD Barcelona Children's Hospital, Universitat de Barcelona, Barcelona, Spain
e-mail: apastego44@alumnes.ub.edu; lucas.krauel@sjd.es

L. Krauel (ed.), *Survival Handbook in Pediatric Surgical Oncology*,
https://doi.org/10.1007/978-3-031-65890-7_8

inguinal zone). In the supraclavicular region, any palpable lymph node should raise the suspicion of severe disease, because this finding is associated with cancer in about 25% for patients under the age of 40 [3].

In terms of classification, we can use time criteria for dividing it as acute (less than 2 weeks of evolution), subacute (2–6 weeks), and chronic (more than 6 weeks); also, by location, lymphadenopathy could appear in one single region (localized) or presenting as generalized when it appears in two or more noncontiguous regions [4].

8.2 Benign Findings

As we said, the presence of enlarged lymph nodes is not infrequent and often is related with signs and symptoms that explain its growth. It is important to note that about 40% of children between 2 and 5 years of age and about 90% of children of 4–8 years of age will have a palpable lymph node [3], most of which will be painless and self-limited.

Viral upper respiratory diseases are the most frequent cause of lymphadenopathy in children and often are accompanied by cervical enlarged lymph nodes, following lymph node chains, usually bilateral, with no tenderness, and nonadherent to deep tissues. This lymphadenopathy is self-limited, remitting with the virosis or after a few days [1].

When the etiology is bacterial, involved lymph nodes are near the site of infection, and looks swell, tender, and fluctuant, with inflammatory changes of the skin surrounding it (this condition is also known as lymphadenitis). In general, *Streptococcus* and *Staphylococcus* lymphadenitis are localized, with no systemic lymph node enlargements. Odontogenic origin could generate a similar clinical picture in children [5].

Lymphadenopathy of benign origin will resolve spontaneously in most cases, or with specific treatment/drainage if a bacterial infection is present. An acceptable time to wait is 2 weeks, but if there are no signs or symptoms of concern, the pediatric team could maintain an expectant conduct for another 1–2 weeks, before performing laboratory tests, starting an antibiotic course, or considering surgical consultation, on a case-by-case basis, which may depend on multiple factors [6].

An extensive and detailed approach to benign conditions that generate lymphadenopathy and their management are beyond the scope of this chapter.

8.3 Specific Findings

Taking into consideration that lymphadenopathy is a common condition in children, with an infrequent but worrisome number of cases which is a sign of severe disease, we should keep tools at hand to raise suspicion and decide to perform invasive procedures for obtaining a diagnosis [2]. However, several "alarming findings" (Table 8.2) should warranty a fast evaluation and study, usually including a biopsy, because these signs, symptoms, and laboratory/imaging findings have risk to be associated with cancer [4].

If there are no alarming findings, it's necessary to perform a detailed exploration of the patient, searching for an explanation that could elucidate the origin of the lymph node enlargement.

8.3.1 History

- Timing: When lymphadenopathy remains or grows after 1–2 weeks, the pediatric team could start an antibiotic course and/or perform laboratory tests. In this scenario, if the diagno-

Table 8.2 Alarming findings [3, 4]

Supraclavicular lymph nodes
Generalized lymphadenopathy
Systemic symptoms (weight loss >10%, night sweats, fever >7 days)
Nontender >2 cm lymph nodes that remain or grow after 2-week antibiotic course
Nontender >1 cm lymph nodes with onset in neonatal period
Abnormalities in chest radiography (mediastinal mass) or complete blood count (two or more cytopenia), elevated LDH/ESR/CRP

LDH lactate dehydrogenase, *ESR* erythrocyte sedimentation rate, *CRP* C-reactive protein

sis hasn't been found and there are no clinical changes after 2–4 weeks, then biopsy should be considered [6].

- Behavior and contacts: History of kitten scratches, close contact with ill people, sexual habits in adolescents, recent travels, or a suspicion of sexual abuse could become helpful in the diagnostic approach of lymphadenopathy. The absence of that also would warrant a biopsy [3].
- Clinical history: Autoimmune disorders, history of malignancy, hematologic diseases, and other chronic conditions could be the source of lymphadenopathy.
- Systemic symptoms: Clinical manifestations that could explain a lymph node enlargement could be a rush, arthralgias, upper respiratory symptoms, dental pain, and many others.

8.3.2 Physical Examination

- General: A thorough evaluation should be performed, including weight. Findings like conjunctivitis, throat enanthem, ear suppuration, or gingivitis could explain cervical lymphadenopathy; cardiopulmonary examination could reveal a mediastinal mass, and abdomen palpation could reveal a hepatomegaly or splenomegaly [4].
- Lymph node: We need to consider several aspects of lymphadenopathy when palpating. Despite the size and location previously discussed, another important characteristic is consistency, especially when palpating a rubbery, large, irregular, and fixed mass or conglomerate [2].

8.4 Further Study

If necessary, laboratory tests are made according to the diagnostic suspicion, looking for evaluation of general status (complete blood count, coagulation tests, biochemical tests, etc.) and/or searching for a specific etiology (viral serology, cultures, polymerase chain reaction test, antibodies, among others). The need for these tests is decided by the pediatric team.

Table 8.3 Ultrasonographic signs of concern [2, 3, 5]

Distorted architecture
Hypervascularity
Loss of central hilum, echogenicity of hilum
Irregular borders
Sonographic heterogeneity

Imaging tests can be requested for characterization of lymphadenopathy. Ultrasound is the most useful tool, and several findings could indicate the presence of severe disease (Table 8.3) [2, 3, 5]. This study is also useful for determining the exact location, number, and size of lymph nodes if there exists the possibility of a biopsy.

Other imaging tests, like computed tomography (CT)-scan or MRI, are requested to rule out solid masses, metastasis, or other conditions.

8.5 Biopsy

The moment and the indications for performing a biopsy are diffuse, but a good approximation to the latter is the conditions resumed in Table 8.2. When we have the presence of one or more of the alarming findings, a biopsy should be warranted.

At this stage, determining the need for a cutdown is more difficult to establish with certainty, as the etiology of lymphadenopathy can be insidious, such as in cases of tuberculosis or infections like Epstein-Barr virus or cytomegalovirus, where diagnosis is often slow and challenging. Other times it's necessary to wait for the effects of an antibiotic course, like in *Bartonella henselae* infections. In general, however, if there is no definitive etiology after 4–6 weeks, lymphadenopathy is stable or grows, and if an attempt of treatment is ineffective, a biopsy should be warranted [1].

It's important to remark that communication within the pediatric team is crucial for obtaining a diagnosis at the correct timing, without repeated or missing tests.

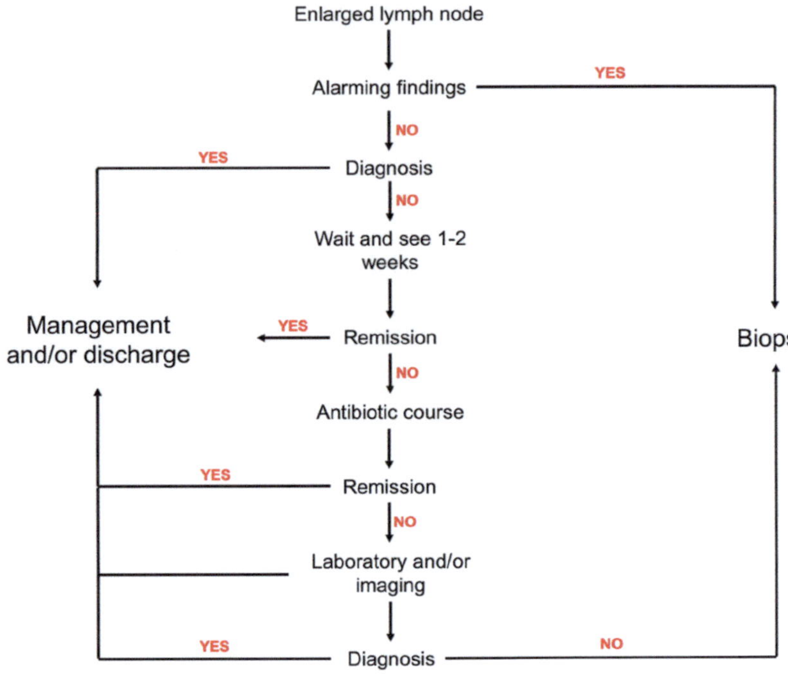

Fig. 8.1 General algorithm for lymph node enlargement course of action

Figure 8.1 shows a general algorithm that we propose to follow.

8.6 Performing a Lymph Node Biopsy

The first step is to choose which lymph node will be the right one. The largest, hardest and/or most tender should be selected, considering its accessibility, too. In cases of generalized lymphadenopathy and similar lymph nodes, the order of selection is supraclavicular, cervical, axillary, and inguinal [3]. Careful physical examination and thorough analysis of imaging are useful and should be performed.

If the patient has a mediastinal mass, it's important to request an anesthesia evaluation, to determine whether it might be necessary to take additional measures in the operating room or consider the use of sedation without intubation [6].

For the surgical approach, we recommend performing an excisional biopsy whenever possible, as it preserves the complete, unaltered architecture of the lymph node, allowing for a more thorough and accurate pathological examination. Careful dissection of the node is necessary to prevent accidental damage to vascular, nervous, or other vital structures. Gentle handling of the node is essential (a suture can be used for traction), and the hilum should be ligated before excision to avoid lymphatic leakage. When the mass is like a conglomerate and is not possible to identify a single node, is an option to make an incisional biopsy taking at least one sample of 1 cm^3.

A core biopsy could be another option when lymph nodes are inaccessible, like retroperitoneal location. Ultrasound guidance improves performance of this technique, obtaining similar results to excisional biopsy [3]; therefore, the help of the radiology team is crucial to obtain a good sample.

The sample should be sent to pathology as a fresh specimen, unless otherwise decided after a multidisciplinary agreement on a case-by-case basis [2].

8.7 Complications

Bleeding could be a problem if the surgical field involves major vessels, like in cervical lymph nodes. A thorough knowledge of anatomy and careful dissection should diminish the risk. Nerve injury in the neck and axilla is another complication that could be reduced with the latter considerations [2].

Infection is rare because this type of surgical intervention is usually clean.

A seroma can occur if lymph leak is not prevented. Control and ligation of hilum minimize this possibility. Bipolar and sealing devices can be helpful.

Probably, one of the worst complications is not surgical but to obtain an insufficient sample. It's frustrating to perform a second procedure and delay diagnosis and treatment, especially if malignancy is suspected. To reduce this scenario, it is crucial to perform a thorough physical examination and request imaging if necessary.

Surgeon's Checklist

1. Verify if the patient has a thorough study, and complete it if it's insufficient (coordinate with pediatric team).
2. Perform a careful physical examination to choose the best lymph node to sample, and request an ultrasound if you need orientation.
3. Consider surgical biopsy if the patient has one or more alarming findings.
4. If the suspicion is a lymphoproliferative disorder, check or request a chest X-ray to rule out mediastinal mass. If present, inform anesthesia before proceeding.
5. Review your anatomy area before operating, especially in cervical and axillary enlarged lymph nodes.
6. Mark the site of incision on the overlying skin, assure a good exposure, and seek to take a complete lymph node.
7. The sample should be sent as a fresh specimen.
8. Make sure you coordinate all required studies; pathology, microbiology, polymerase chain reaction (PCR), and molecular (best if you distribute the samples).

References

1. Farndon S, Behjati S, Jonas N, Messahel B. How to use… lymph node biopsy in paediatrics. Arch Dis Child Educ Pract Ed. 2017;102(5):244–8.
2. Baerg J, Pepper VK, Munoz AN. Lymphadenopathy. Pediatric Surgery NAT. 2021.
3. Grant CN, Aldrink J, Lautz TB, Tracy ET, Rhee DS, Baertschiger RM, et al. Lymphadenopathy in children: a streamlined approach for the surgeon—a report from the APSA Cancer Committee. J Pediatr Surg. 2021;56:274–81.
4. Soldes OS, Younger JG, Hirschl RB. Predictors of malignancy in childhood peripheral lymphadenopathy. J Pediatr Surg. 1999;34(10):1447–52.
5. Locke R, Comfort R, Kubba H. When does an enlarged cervical lymph node in a child need excision? A systematic review. Int J Pediatr Otorhinolaryngol. 2014;78:393–401.
6. de Campos Vieira Abib S, Chui CH, Cox S, Abdelhafeez AH, Fernandez-Pineda I, Elgendy A, et al. International Society of Paediatric Surgical Oncology (IPSO) surgical practice guidelines. Ecancermedicalscience. 2022;16:1356.

9 Surgical Incisions in Pediatric Surgical Oncology

Emily Christison-Lagay

The surgical treatment of pediatric cancer is a complex, multidisciplinary process aimed at optimizing outcomes and minimizing complications and must take into account the questions of **what** procedure to perform, **when** to perform it, and **how** to approach resection (Surgical Checklist). Choosing an optimal approach for resecting a tumor is a **critical** first step to a successful resection. An incision that limits exposure to the necessary field of resection will be associated with both poorer outcomes and more complications. For instance, the approach to a neuroblastoma which partially encases the aorta, celiac, and superior mesenteric artery roots will be facilitated by a thoracoabdominal approach which allows access to the proximal and distal aorta. Similarly, while minimally invasive approaches (MIS) are increasingly applied, the surgeon choosing this approach must be confident that an MIS approach offers an equivalent oncologic resection [1]. Data from lymph node resections obtained during laparoscopic resection of Wilms' tumor suggest that lymph node yield is lower than with open cases with some patients not undergoing any lymph node sampling, potentially leading to tumor under-staging [2, 3]. Common incisions to tumors in the neck, chest, abdomen, and pelvis are described below as a preliminary guide to a surgical approach (Table 9.1).

Table 9.1 Tumor type with common incisional approach

Tumor	Approach
Thyroid	Transverse cervical
Thymus	Transverse cervical, thoracoscopic resection, sternotomy
Lateral neck lymph nodes	Extended cervical incision
Mediastinal neuroblastoma	Trap door, thoracoscopic resection
Pleuropulmonary blastoma	Posterior lateral thoracotomy, thoracoscopic resection (small)
Anterior mediastinal mass	Posterior lateral thoracotomy, sternotomy, thoracoscopic resection
Pulmonary neoplasm	Posterior lateral thoracotomy, thoracoscopic resection
Hepatoblastoma	Right-sided subcostal or Chevron incision, robotic or laparoscopic hepatectomy

(continued)

E. Christison-Lagay (✉)
Yale New Haven Children's Hospital, Yale School of Medicine, New Haven, CT, USA
e-mail: emily.christison-lagay@yale.edu

L. Krauel (ed.), *Survival Handbook in Pediatric Surgical Oncology*,
https://doi.org/10.1007/978-3-031-65890-7_9

Table 9.1 (continued)

Tumor	Approach
Wilms' tumor	Transverse abdominal incision, thoracoabdominal incision, laparoscopic or robotic approach (must include lymph node dissection)
Neuroblastoma (sympathetic chain)	Thoracoabdominal incision, transverse abdominal incision
Adrenal mass	Subcostal incision, thoracoabdominal incision, transverse abdominal incision, laparoscopic or robotic approach
Pancreatic head mass	Right subcostal incision, upper midline laparotomy
Pancreatic tail mass	Left subcostal incision, upper midline laparotomy, laparoscopic or robotic approach
Pelvic tumor	Lower midline laparotomy
Ovarian mass	Midline laparotomy, laparoscopic or robotic approach
Testicular mass	Inguinal incision, may be extended to scrotum

9.1 Approaches to Cervical Tumors (Fig. 9.1)

9.1.1 Central Neck Incision

A central neck incision is used to resect thyroid tumors as well as to approach the thymus, lymph nodes of the central neck, or, rarely, the cervical trachea. After placing a transverse scapular roll gently hyperextending the neck, a transverse skin incision is made in a skin crease approximately 2–3 cm (often described as two fingerbreadths) above the clavicle. The incision is carried through the platysma and subplatysmal flaps are raised superior to the level of the hyoid and inferior to the level of the sternal notch. The strap muscles are separated in the midline and retracted laterally to expose the thyroid and trachea. Access to the superior pole may be facilitated by division of the sternothyroid muscle 1–2 cm proximal to its insertion on the thyroid cartilage.

9.1.2 Modified Lateral Neck Dissection

Patients who have evidence of disease in the lateral neck (including metastatic thyroid disease and neuroblastoma) are best approached through incisions that would facilitate a modified lateral neck dissection. A variety of acceptable incisions exist including a longer collar incision (extending laterally from a central neck incision to the posterior boundary of the sternocleidomastoid) or a "hockey stick" incision which begins as a transverse surgical incision and curves cephalad crossing the muscle belly of the sternocleidomastoid extending superiorly to approximately 3 cm below the earlobe. A "T"- or "I"-shaped incision with a high transverse component along the j line and a vertical component along the sternocleidomastoid is not typically required. As with the transverse cervical incision, exposure to underlying lymph nodes and the vascular and nerve structures in the lateral neck is facilitated by the construction of generous subplatysmal flaps.

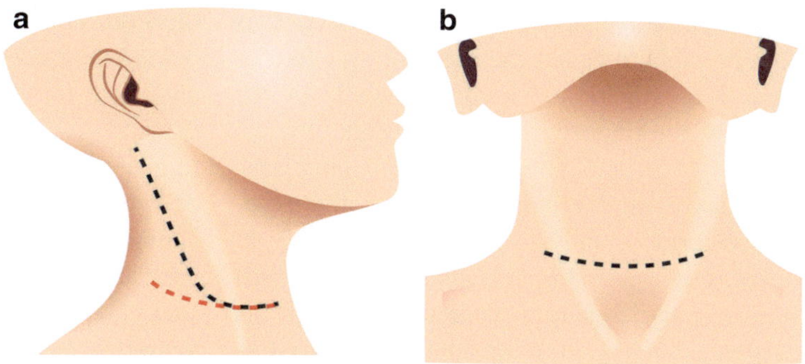

Fig. 9.1 Neck incisions. (**a**) Lateral incisions for modified radical dissection. (**b**) Transverse neck incision. (Figures courtesy of K. Christison-Lagay)

9.2 Trap Door Approach to Tumors of the Cervicothoracic Junction (Fig. 9.2)

Tumors of the cervicothoracic junction and apical thoracic tumors encroaching upon the great vessels or brachial plexus are often best approached through an incision that permits access structures of the neck and chest [4]. The patient is placed supine with a roll beneath the shoulders, the arm ipsilateral to the lesion outstretched, and the contralateral arm tucked. Anesthesia is induced, preferably with a double-lumen endotracheal tube or a single-lumen endotracheal tube with a bronchial blocker. The head is then rotated 30°–45° away from the side of the tumor. A transverse incision is begun superior and parallel to the clavicle (or along the anterior border of the sternocleidomastoid with a descending course if access is needed to the structures of the neck) to the midportion of the suprasternal notch, continued downward through the midline sternum to the fifth interspace, and then laterally through the fifth interspace to the anterior axillary line. The pectoralis is divided close to its point of insertion and the intercostal muscles divided at the fifth interspace. The pleura is entered, and the internal mammary vessels are isolated, ligated, and divided. The retrosternal space is bluntly dissected, and a sternal saw is used to divide the sternum to the level of the fifth interspace and then laterally to the thoracotomy. Bleeding from the edge of the sternum is treated with bone wax. The sternal and a portion of the clavicular head of the sternocleidomastoid are divided close to their points of origin and marked with sutures for later approximation. The strap muscles are similarly divided. A Finochietto retractor is then placed between the cut edges of the sternum allowing excellent exposure.

For large anterior mediastinal masses that require less exposure of the great vessels, a fifth intercostal space anterior thoracotomy (as described above) may be sufficient. The extraction of a large mass may be facilitated by division of the sixth (and seventh) rib in the anterior axillary line, allowing the inferior hemithorax to swing away from the spine. The ribs can be reapproximated at the end of the procedure.

9.3 Approaches to Thoracic Tumors (Fig. 9.2)

9.3.1 Thoracotomy

When an open approach is needed for tumors of the thoracic cavity, including those originating from the lung parenchyma or tracheobronchial tree as well as the anterior and posterior mediastinum, a posterolateral thoracotomy incision is frequently chosen. The patient is placed in a full lateral decubitus position with lateral stabilization and protection of neurovascular structures with an axillary roll. A skin incision is made 2–3 cm below the scapular tip. Classically the incision is described as curving from below the nipple to a vertical line halfway between the spinous processes and the medial scapular edge requiring division of the latissimus dorsi (and sometimes serratus anterior) muscle; however, this extent of incision is rarely necessary. It is often possible to center the incision over the triangle of auscultation (bounded medially by the border of the trapezius, laterally by the vertical scapular edge, and inferiorly by the latissimus dorsi), sweeping the latissimus anteriorly, trapezius posteriorly, and requiring division only of the intercostal muscles. It is also possible to perform a muscle-sparing approach through an incision extending from the anterior axillary line to 2 cm below the scapular tip, sweeping the latissimus posteriorly and mobilizing the serratus off the chest wall.

Alternatively, some surgeons prefer a vertical axillary muscle-sparing thoracotomy incision. With the patient placed in a lateral decubitus position and the ipsilateral arm maximally abducted and flexed at the elbow, a 5–7 cm skin incision is placed posterior to lateral edge of the pectoralis major beginning around the level of the third rib. After coming through the subcutaneous tissue, the pectoralis is mobilized laterally, freeing it off the chest wall, and the serratus anterior is reflected posteriorly by mobilizing its insertions on the fourth and fifth rib. Once in the pleural cavity, the intercostal muscles are divided as far posteriorly as possible.

9.3.2 Clamshell

Large mediastinal tumors which require access to both hemithoraces are best approached through a bilateral anterior thoracotomy or "clamshell" incision. The patient is placed supine with a roll behind the midportion of the chest. The arms are abducted to 90° at the shoulder and elbow. General anesthesia is induced with a double-lumen or single-lumen endotracheal tube capable of lung isolation. An anterior curvilinear incision is made along the fifth interspace bilaterally from each anterior axillary line, connecting at the midline. The pleura is entered, and the mammary vessels are isolated, ligated, and divided. The retrosternal space is then bluntly dissected and the sternum divided transversely with a sternal saw. A Finochietto retractor is placed, allowing for exposure of both pleural cavities, from the pulmonary hilum to the posterior aspect of the diaphragm.

9.3.3 Sternotomy

A sternotomy is often the incision of choice for the resection of anterior mediastinal tumors including teratomas, mediastinal germ cell tumors, and large thymic masses [5]. The patient is placed supine on the operating room table, and a skin incision is made in the midline from the sternal notch just inferior to the xiphoid process. The subcutaneous tissue is divided with electrocautery and the sternal periosteum incised. A finger is placed in the sternal notch to free the posterior aspect of the sternum and sweep the pleura aside. The lungs are deflated, and a reciprocating sternal saw is used to divide the sternum. Bleeding along the ster-

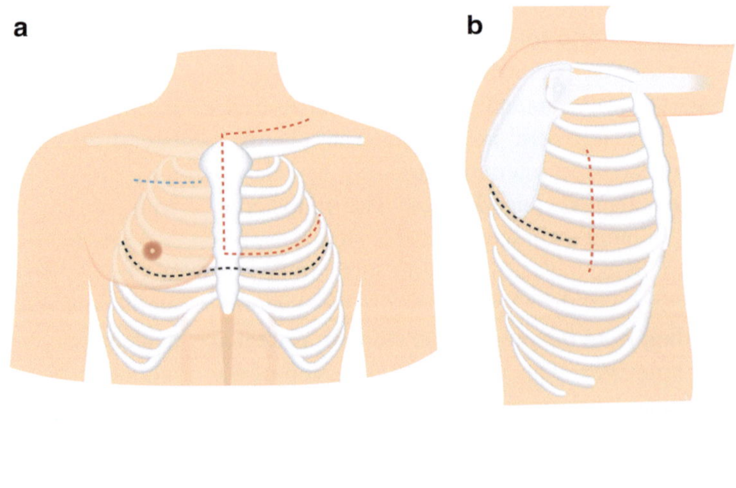

Fig. 9.2 Thoracic incisions. (**a**) (Blue dashed line) Chamberlain; (Red dashed line) Trapdoor; (Black dashed line) clam shell. (**b**) (Black dashed line) Posterior lateral; (Red dashed line) vertical axillary. (Figures courtesy of K. Christison-Lagay)

nal edge can be controlled by electrocautery or bone wax. For large, unilateral anterior mediastinal tumors which extend to the midline, it is often possible to combine a sternotomy with a hemi-clamshell incision to gain necessary exposure.

9.3.4 Chamberlain Procedure

While thoracoscopy has largely supplanted open biopsy of lymphadenopathy in the anterior mediastinum, the Chamberlain procedure remains an excellent option for patients who may not tolerate a general anesthetic and are sufficiently mature to undergo a procedure under light sedation. A 3–4 cm incision is made beginning 1 cm lateral to the sternal border in the second or third rib space and deepened through the subcutaneous tissue and pectoralis muscles to expose the extrapleural mediastinum. In larger patients, the second, third, or fourth costal cartilage may be resected to aid in exposure.

9.3.5 Chest Wall Resections

For masses originating off the chest wall, the patient is typically placed in the lateral decubitus position as for a standard thoracotomy. An exception may be made for anterior tumors in which better access may be achieved with the patient in a prone position. Unlike for primary lung resections, a muscle-sparing approach should not be used as it is necessary to gain wide exposure to the chest wall (and in some cases, en bloc resection of muscle may be needed to achieve negative margins). It is always good practice to ensure that any involved lung can be safely resected prior to initiating the chest wall resection. Assessment of the lung and often the extent of chest wall involvement may be facilitated by thoracoscopy prior to thoracotomy. Local recurrence is minimized by resection of at least one and sometimes two ribs above and below the lesion. It is usually easier to begin with anterior division of the rib with subsequent ligation of the intercostal bundle. Posteriorly, it may be necessary to disarticulate the rib from the transverse process and vertebral body.

Tumors originating from the posterior superior chest wall or involving the structures of the thoracic outlet may be approached through a vertical extension of a (non-muscle-sparing) thoracotomy. This extension is directed cephalad toward C7 along a vertical axis positioned halfway between the medial border of the scapula and the midline spinous processes [6]. The trapezius is divided and the scapula lifted off the chest wall. The insertion of the posterior scalene on the second rib is divided, and the anterior and middle scalene muscles are retracted off the first rib, exposing the brachial plexus and subclavian vessels above the first rib.

9.3.6 Minimally Invasive Approaches

Many resections of pulmonary tumors may be achieved through minimally invasive (thoracoscopic or robotic) techniques with the patient in a lateral decubitus position. These typically employ three or four 5 mm thoracoscopic trocars, with the trocar for the camera placed in the anterior axillary line of the fifth interspace. Working ports are typically placed in the midaxillary line of the fourth to eighth interspace depending upon surgeon preference and optimizing triangulation for dissection of the pulmonary vascular structures, with a fourth port placed posteriorly (if necessary) for additional retraction. Specimens are removed via the inferior-most port which can be enlarged if necessary.

The thymus may also be approached thoracoscopically through either the right or left chest with the patient in a supine position with a small bump under the ipsilateral side of trocar placement and the arms abducted [7, 8]. Three 5 mm trocars are placed: the anterior-midaxillary line of the third interspace, the posterior axillary line of the fifth interspace, and the anterior axillary line of the fourth interspace. Occasionally a fourth port is placed in the midclavicular line of the sixth or seventh interspace to help with retraction.

9.4 Approaches to Abdominal and Retroperitoneal Tumors (Fig. 9.3)

9.4.1 Midline Abdominal Laparotomy Incision

A midline abdominal incision provides excellent exposure to most of the abdomen and central retroperitoneum and is the incision of choice for open procedures on the intestines, pelvis (including malignant ovarian masses), retroperitoneal lymph nodes, and, often, the pancreas. The extent of the incision is governed by the size and location of the tumor and should stay centered on the linea alba.

9.4.2 Transverse Abdominal Incision

In young patients in whom the ratio of the vertical diameter to the transverse diameter of the abdomen is close to 1 (typically children <5 years of age), large tumors are often approached via a transverse rather than a vertical incision. This includes the standard approach to Wilms' tumors and, in many institutions, neuroblastoma. The length of the incision depends upon the size of the tumor but typically extends from the mid- to anterior axillary line and crosses the midline approximately two fingerbreadths above the umbilicus. The incision should be long enough to permit full abdominal exploration.

9.4.3 Subcostal Incision

Most hepatic resections can be approached by a right subcostal incision ("Kocher incision") or a bilateral subcostal incision with a vertical extension ("Chevron incision"). This is also an optimal incision for an anterior approach to the adrenal. The patient is placed supine with the right arm extended and abducted to 90°. Some surgeons prefer a small vertical roll under the right flank permitting incisional access to the posterior axillary line. The incision is placed parallel to and approximately 4 cm below the costal margin. In patients with a narrow costal arch, the incision may be extended cephalad toward the xiphoid in the midline. Superior extension via median sternotomy is also possible and allows access to the supradiaphragmatic vena cava and may improve exposure of the hepatic veins if necessary. Large right-sided posterior tumors or those in which there is inferior vena caval (IVC) extension of venous thrombosis may be better approached through a right-sided thoracoabdominal incision (see below).

9.4.4 Thoracoabdominal Incision

A thoracoabdominal incision provides unparalleled access to the vascular structures of the retroperitoneum and is often the incision of choice for neuroblastoma with image define risk factors and some Wilms' tumors (especially large right-sided tumors with IVC clot extension) [9]. The

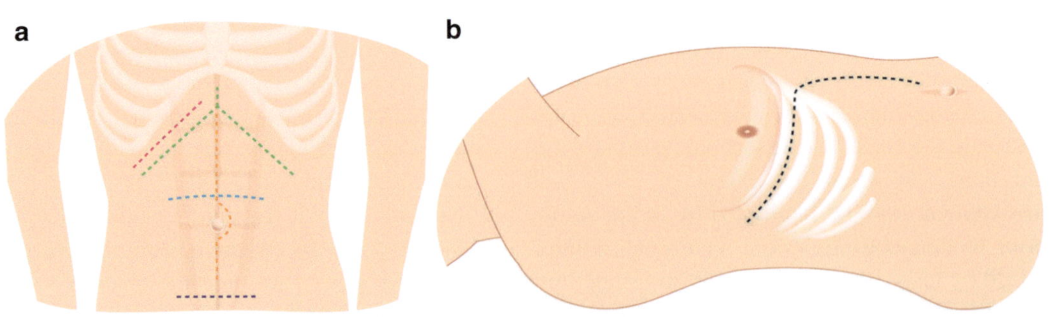

Fig. 9.3 Abdominal incisions. (**a**) (Pink dashed line) Subcostal/"Kocher"; (Green dashed line) Chevron; (Orange dashed line) midline; (Blue dashed line) transverse; (Purple dashed line) Pfannenstiel; (**b**) (Black dashed line) Thoracoabdominal. (Figures courtesy of K. Christison-Lagay)

patient is placed in a lazy (30°–45°) lateral position, often best achieved with a beanbag generating lateral thoracic flexion. The exact position and length of the incision are determined by the tumor to be removed. A neuroblastoma confined to the upper or mid-abdomen may be approached through a 6–8 cm incision centered over the tenth rib (entering the ninth intercostal space) beginning at the midaxillary line and extending onto the abdominal wall; if pelvic access is necessary, the incision may be extended to the midline and then curved down along the linea alba. If access is needed into the mid-thoracic cavity, this incision can be moved cephalad to the seventh interspace. If the deep incision is centered upon the inferior rib of the interspace, the intercostal muscles can be preserved along with their vascular supply and innervation. The incision should expose both the peritoneal cavity and pleural space prior to division of the costal margin. Following division of the costal margin, the diaphragm is divided along its lateral margin, approximately 2 cm off the junction with the chest wall. This provides a large enough "cuff" for diaphragmatic reapproximation during closure while preserving phrenic nerve innervation to the body of the muscle. Some surgeons like to place stay sutures in the diaphragm prior to division to facilitate eventual realignment during closure.

9.4.5 Minimally Invasive Approaches to Abdominal or Retroperitoneal Tumors

Because many intra-abdominal or retroperitoneal tumors are either very large in size or associated with image-defined risk factors which might complicate a minimally invasive approach, open approaches are often preferred. Nonetheless, laparoscopic and robotic resections may be attempted if the surgeon feels that an equivalent resection is possible. This includes approaches to liver, adrenal, renal, pancreatic, and ovarian neoplasms as well as to lymph node dissections of the retroperitoneum. Suggested port placements are described below with the caveat that there is considerable variability among described approaches. Once fully mobilized the specimen may be retrieved via a small incision (hand port, upper midline, paraumbilical, or Pfannenstiel).

Left adrenalectomy, nephrectomy, or distal pancreatectomy: The patient is placed in a lazy lateral position, with the elevation of the left side to approximately 45°–60°. Four 5 mm ports are used: an umbilical port, a subcostal port in the midclavicular line, a subcostal port in the anterior axillary line, and fourth port bisecting the two subcostal ports at or below the level of the umbilicus. If the renal vessels are divided with a stapler, one of the lateral ports can be enlarged to allow passage of the stapling device.

Right adrenalectomy or nephrectomy: The patient is positioned as previously described for a left adrenalectomy. The ports are placed in mirror image with the addition of a fifth 5 mm port for liver retraction in the left epigastrium.

Retroperitoneal lymph node dissection: Many adult uro-oncologists perform robotic retroperitoneal lymph node dissections (often in combination with nephrectomy or partial nephrectomy), and this has been successfully described in pediatric patients as well [10]. The patient is placed in a modified lateral decubitus position with the table flexed. An 8 mm midline robotic trocar is placed at about the level of the 11th rib. Three additional midline 8 mm robotic trocars are then placed in a linear configuration as well as a periumbilical 12 mm AirSeal port. A 5 mm left upper quadrant (LUQ) port is used for liver retraction for right-sided tumors. Alternatively, this dissection can be performed in the supine position with five trocars (four 8 mm trocars equally spaced along a transverse line at the level of the anterior superior iliac spine (ASIS) and a five 12 mm assistant trocar in the right lower abdomen half the distance to the pubis from the line of trocars) or six trocars (two 8 mm trocars just medial to the ASIS bilaterally, an 8 mm trocar along the left anterior axillary line midway between the costal margin and the ASIS, a 12 mm camera trocar placed in the midline 5 cm below the umbilicus, and 5 and 12 mm assistant ports along the right anterior axillary line at the costal margin and midway between the costal margin and the ASIS, respectively). The patient is then placed in 20° Trendelenburg and the table tilted right or left.

Hepatic resections: Both laparoscopic and robotic approaches to liver resection have been widely applied in adult populations, but the adoption of these approaches in children has been limited to large centers and high-volume surgeons [11]. As such, these approaches should be utilized only if sufficient experience of the surgeon allows safe conduct. In general, four or five trocars are used. One approach describes a right paraumbilical camera port, right subcostal port, left epigastric port, left lateral subcostal port, and a right lower quadrant port in the midclavicular line. Many other configurations have been described including three ports along the right costal margin, a 5 mm port along the left costal margin in the midclavicular line, and an umbilical port.

Surgeon's Checklist

1. Confirm diagnosis, laterality, and oncologic protocol requirements for procedure (margins, lymph node dissection or sampling, need for additional tissue sampling, incorporation of previous biopsy tracts into resection).
2. Confirm tumor stage and ensure that this does not affect choice of operation.
3. Review imaging and anatomy: what critical structures may be in the operative field, and what is the plan for preserving these intraoperatively? Is nerve monitoring needed? What is the plan for vascular control? Will ureteral stenting be helpful?
4. Mark out incision and any previous incisions. Decide whether resection can proceed safely through previous incision? If exposure is insufficient, plan next step (larger incision?)
5. Define criteria which would guide a switch from a minimally invasive approach to an open approach. An MIS approach should never jeopardize oncologic outcomes.
6. Check labwork including metabolic profile, complete blood count, and coagulation panel. Check von Willebrand factor (vWF) in Wilms' tumor patients. Have cross-matched blood, platelets, and plasma available if necessary.
7. Review plan with anesthesiology team and nursing team. Ensure that you have the correct instruments.

References

1. Ezekian B, Englum BR, Gulack BC, Rialon KL, Kim J, Talbot LJ, et al. Comparing oncologic outcomes after minimally invasive and open surgery for pediatric neuroblastoma and Wilms tumor. Pediatr Blood Cancer. 2018;65(1).
2. Warmann SW, Godzinski J, van Tinteren H, Heij H, Powis M, Sandstedt B, et al. Minimally invasive nephrectomy for Wilms tumors in children—data from SIOP 2001. J Pediatr Surg. 2014;49(11):1544–8.
3. Romao RL, Weber B, Gerstle JT, Grant R, Pippi Salle JL, Bägli DJ, et al. Comparison between laparoscopic and open radical nephrectomy for the treatment of primary renal tumors in children: single-center experience over a 5-year period. J Pediatr Urol. 2014;10(3):488–94.
4. Christison-Lagay ER, Darcy DG, Stanelle EJ, Dasilva S, Avila E, La Quaglia MP. "Trap-door" and "clamshell" surgical approaches for the management of pediatric tumors of the cervicothoracic junction and mediastinum. J Pediatr Surg. 2014;49(1):172–176; discussion 176–7.
5. Miller VM, Disharoon M, Padilla LA, Beierle EA, Dabal RJ. A multidisciplinary surgical approach to mediastinal masses in children. World J Pediatr Congenit Heart Surg. 2023;14(2):180–4.
6. Rea F, Marulli G, Sartori F. Posterior-lateral (Shaw-Paulson) approach to Pancoast tumor. CTSnet2011.
7. Christison-Lagay E, Dharia B, Vajsar J, Kim PC. Efficacy and safety of thoracoscopic thymectomy in the treatment of juvenile myasthenia gravis. Pediatr Surg Int. 2013;29(6):583–6.
8. Derderian SC, Potter DD, Bansal S, Rowse PG, Partrick DA. Open versus thoracoscopic thymectomy for juvenile myasthenia gravis. J Pediatr Surg. 2020;55(9):1850–3.
9. Ross SL, Greenwald BM, Howell JD, Pon S, Rutigliano DN, Spicyn N, et al. Outcomes following thoracoabdominal resection of neuroblastoma. Pediatr Crit Care Med. 2009;10(6):681–6.
10. Garg H, Mansour AM, Psutka SP, Kim SP, Porter J, Gaspard CS, et al. Robot-assisted retroperitoneal lymph node dissection: a systematic review of perioperative outcomes. BJU Int. 2023;132(1):9–30.
11. Rayman S, Sucandy I, Ross SB, Crespo K, Syblis C, Rosemurgy A. A propensity score matched analysis of robotic and open hepatectomy for treatment of liver tumors. Clinical outcomes, oncological survival, and costs comparison. J Robot Surg. 2023;17:2399.

10 Renal Tumors

Simone de Campos Vieira Abib
and Hafeez Abdelhafeez

10.1 Introduction

- Wilms tumor (WT) is the second most frequent solid tumor in children after neuroblastoma. They represent 6% of all childhood cancers and are the most common renal tumor, accounting for 85% of renal tumor patients less than 15 years of age [1].
- Ten percent of cases are associated with congenital anomalies or predisposition syndromes: Wilms tumor, aniridia, genitourinary malformations, and a range of mental disabilities (WAGR) syndrome, Denys-Drash syndrome, and Beckwith-Wiedemann syndrome, among others.
- Five to 7% of Wilms tumor cases are bilateral and can be synchronous or metachronous.
- Vascular extension occurs in 15% of cases, mostly to the renal vein. Extension to the vena cava and right atrium occurs in 4% of cases [2–6].
- Non-Wilms tumors (renal cell carcinoma, rhabdoid tumor of the kidney, clear cell sarcoma, congenital mesoblastic nephroma, multilocular cystic nephroma, renal medullary carcinoma) are rarer and will usually be diagnosed after nephrectomy.
- Other kidney malignant tumors: primary renal synovial sarcoma, anaplastic sarcoma of the kidney, primary renal myoepithelial carcinoma, Primitive neuroectodermal tumor (PNET), Ewing sarcoma of the kidney, lymphoma (usually affects both kidneys), and neuroblastoma.
- Pathologies mimicking renal tumors: xanthogranulomatous pyelonephritis and trauma.

10.2 Diagnosis

10.2.1 Clinical Presentation

- Healthy child with asymptomatic abdominal mass. Some cases can present hematuria, hypertension, spontaneous bleeding, or incidentally when image investigation is made for trauma.
- Abdominal pain is associated with tumor rupture or bleeding, anaplasia, and higher stages.
- Stigmata of associated syndromes should be observed: aniridia, hemihypertrophy, somatic overgrowth, clinical manifestations of Beckwith-Wiedemann syndrome, and genitourinary anomalies including disorders of sexual development, hypospadias, and cryptorchidism.

S. de Campos Vieira Abib (✉)
Pediatric Oncology Institute—GRAACC, Federal University of São Paulo, São Paulo, Brazil

H. Abdelhafeez
St Jude Research Hospital, Memphis, TN, USA
e-mail: Hafeez.abdelhafeez@stjude.org

L. Krauel (ed.), *Survival Handbook in Pediatric Surgical Oncology*,
https://doi.org/10.1007/978-3-031-65890-7_10

10.2.2 Labs

10.2.2.1 Complete Blood and Metabolic Profiles

*Caution: 5% of Wilms tumor cases have acquired von Willebrand phenomenon with severe coagulopathy. This should be considered in the preoperative phase for catheter implantation.

10.2.3 Imaging

1. Ultrasound: determines the origin of the tumor (kidney) and evaluates vascular extension (its level and if there is blood flow around it or not).
2. Contrasted dual-phase CT scan or MRI of the abdomen and pelvis: the claw sign suggests a renal tumor.
3. Non-contrast CT chest is recommended for accurate staging and adequate therapy intensification.

10.2.3.1 Checklist for Surgical Planning [7]

1. Evaluation of findings suggestive of WT or other differential diagnoses such as Diffuse hyperplastic perilobar nephroblastomatosis (DHPN) and neuroblastoma.
2. Relation of the renal tumor with surrounding organs and vascular structures.
3. Evaluation of preoperative tumor rupture and signs of abdominal dissemination and pulmonary metastasis.
4. Assessment of cystic areas that are prone to intraoperative rupture.
5. Evaluation of bilateral disease (5%) or coexisting urinary malformations (e.g., single or horseshoe kidney).
6. Evaluation of intravascular extension. If present, assessment of the level and presence or absence of blood flow around it and response to chemotherapy.
7. Evaluation of tumor response and pulmonary metastasis response to chemotherapy.

10.2.4 Perioperative Principles and Staging

- A typical age and imaging findings will *not* require a diagnostic biopsy. The typical age of diagnosis for WT is more than 6 months and less than 7 years.
- Tissue diagnosis (nephrectomy, if feasible; or biopsy) is required to plan therapy for patients who present at an atypical age or have atypical imaging features.
- There are two main protocols to treat patients with WT: Children's Oncology Group (COG) and the International Society of Paediatric Oncology (SIOP). Both protocols report similar survival results. The difference between the two protocols is the use of preoperative chemotherapy (SIOP) or upfront surgery (COG). Both protocols recommend upfront resection for patients less than 6 months of age, because of the relatively higher incidence of congenital mesoblastic nephroma and rhabdoid tumors in this age group (Table 10.1) [8].
- Preoperative chemotherapy is indicated in COG when tumors present with vascular extension above the level of the hepatic veins, bilateral Wilms tumors, gross local invasion that would require en bloc resection of adjacent organs other than the diaphragm and adrenal gland, severe pulmonary compromise from compression by massive tumor or widespread pulmonary metastases, solitary kidney, or the discretion of the operating surgeon that immediate nephrectomy would result in severe morbidity, tumor spill, or incomplete resection.
- SIOP protocol indicates neoadjuvant chemotherapy prior to surgical resection in patients between 6 months and 10 years of age. Typical imaging of Wilms tumors without pathologic confirmation allows the administration of chemotherapy. Patients under 6 months of age are excluded from this approach because there is a higher like-

Table 10.1 Comparison between COG and SIOP protocols

	COG	SIOP
Preoperative chemotherapy	No (only in special situations: bilateral WT, solitary kidney, predisposition syndromes, inferior vena cava tumor thrombus extension to involve the level of hepatic veins, extensive symptomatic pulmonary metastases)	Yes (for renal tumors with typical clinical features)
Staging		
I	• Tumor limited to the kidney and completely resected • No rupture and no biopsy before surgery • No involvement of the renal capsule or renal sinus vessels • Lymph node status is known and negative	• Tumor limited to the kidney or surrounded by a pseudocapsule if outside the normal contour of the kidney • Renal pseudocapsule may be infiltrated but was completely resected and does not reach the outer surface of the kidney • Tumor protrudes into the collecting system/ureter, but does not infiltrate their walls • Intrarenal vessels may be involved • Renal sinus vessels are not involved
II	• Tumor extends beyond the capsule of the kidney and was not completely resected with no evidence of tumor at or beyond the margins of resection • Involvement of renal sinus and renal capsule • Lymph node status is known and negative	• Tumor extends beyond the kidney or penetrates the renal capsule and/or pseudocapsule into the perirenal fat but is completely resected • Tumor infiltrates renal sinus and/or blood and lymphatic renal vessels outside the renal parenchyma but is completely resected • Tumor infiltrates adjacent organs or the vena cava but is completely resected • Tumor has been biopsied (wedge biopsy) before chemotherapy or surgery
III	• Gross macroscopic residual tumor remains after surgery (inoperable, positive surgical margins, tumor spillage surfaces, regional lymph node metastasis, positive peritoneal cytology, transected tumor thrombus) • Tumor rupture • Tumor biopsy before removal	• Incomplete resection of the tumor (gross or microscopic postoperative residual) • Positive lymph nodes • Tumor rupture (pre or intraoperatively) • Tumor penetrated peritoneal surface • Peritoneal tumor implants • Tumor thrombi present at resection • Margins of vessels or ureter transected or removed piecemeal by surgeon
IV	• Hematogenous metastases or lymph node metastases outside the abdomen (e.g., bone, lungs, liver, brain)	• Hematogenous metastases (bone, lungs, liver, brain) or lymph node metastases outside the abdominopelvic region
V	• Bilateral renal tumors at diagnosis. Each side should be staged according to the above classification	• Bilateral renal tumors at diagnosis. Each side should be staged according to the above classification

lihood of an alternate tumor histology such as congenital mesoblastic nephroma that would not be responsive to vincristine and actinomycin-D. Patients above 10 years of age should also be carefully evaluated for non-Wilms tumors as the incidence of renal cell carcinoma increases and up-front resection is more appropriate.

10.2.5 Surgery

10.2.5.1 Surgeon's Checklist

1. *Surgical Planning*
   (a) Multidisciplinary team discussions and planning.
   (b) Evaluation of distant metastases and surrounding organs.

   (c) Evaluation of bilateral disease.
   (d) Evaluation of vascular extension (level and presence of blood flow around the thrombus).
   (e) Evaluation of comorbidities, such as cardiotoxicity due to doxorubicin.
   (f) Response to preoperative chemotherapy (if indicated by protocol of special situations).
   (g) Evaluate capacity of monitoring and anesthesia.
   (h) Safe vascular access.
   (i) Blood sampling.
   (j) Blood bank.
   (k) Postoperative monitoring capacity and pain control.
   (l) If a neoadjuvant chemotherapy protocol is used, surgery should follow blood count recovery, and the planned timing of surgery should not be delayed.
2. *Surgical procedure*

10.3 Wilms Tumor Surgery Checklists

10.3.1 Planning Surgery

- Evaluation of findings suggestive of WT or other differential diagnoses such as DHPN and neuroblastoma or other.
- Relation of the renal tumor with surrounding organs and vascular structures.
- Evaluation of preoperative tumor rupture and signs of abdominal dissemination and pulmonary metastasis.
- Assessment of cystic areas that are prone to intraoperative rupture.
- Evaluation of bilateral disease (5%) or coexisting urinary malformations (e.g., single or horseshoe kidney).
- Evaluation of intravascular extension (10–15%). If present, assessment of the level and presence or absence of blood flow around it, to later assess response to chemotherapy.
- Evaluation of tumor response and pulmonary metastasis response to chemotherapy.
- Multidisciplinary team meeting (MDT) discussion.

10.3.2 Preop

- Review images.
- Assessment of comorbidities.
- Complete blood count and coagulation profile (especially blood count recovery from chemotherapy if indicated preoperatively).
- Blood reserve.
- Calculate and prescribe fasting.
- Check anesthesia availability.
- Check monitoring resources.
- Reliable upper extremity vascular access.
- Appropriate postoperative level of care (ICU if needed).
- Postoperative monitoring.
- Postoperative pain control.

10.3.3 Surgical Steps for Unilateral Tumors

- Transverse of thoracoabdominal incision.
- Depending on the quality of the preoperative images, if there is doubt, access the contralateral kidney to check for bilateral disease. This step is not needed if images are reliable.
- Tumor exposure with colon and/or duodenal medial mobilization.
- Avoid tumor rupture!
- Lateral, superior, and inferior mobilization of the mass.
- Identification of ureter, aorta, or vena cava.
- Intraoperative palpation of Inferior vena cava (IVC) to check image information on intravascular tumor extension.
- Access renal hilum structures and ligate renal artery and vein sequentially.
- Ureter ligation near the bladder.
- En bloc resection of the tumor, with perirenal fat. Rarely are surrounding organs involved and need resection, but if needed, the colon, diaphragm, or pancreatic tail can be resected along with the tumor.
- If the diaphragm is opened, it is safer to place a pleural drain.
- Check if iatrogenic ligation of the contralateral renal vein or superior mesenteric artery

did not occur, especially in huge tumors where the anatomical landmarks are distorted.

- Adequate lymph node sampling (radical lymphadenectomy is not needed; sample lymph nodes from the hilum, periaortic, or pericaval zones, even if they appear normal. Adequate lymph node sampling is crucial! If possible, try to sample approximately seven lymph nodes).
- Adequate documentation of the procedure, including peritoneal seeding, tissue infiltration, lymph node sampling, capsular integrity, and tumor spillage.

Postresection locoregional Radiotherapy (RT) is indicated for patients with stage III disease (when microscopic residual disease is suspected, as in positive lymph node, tumor spillage, or piecemeal resection of the intravascular thrombus) and for stage II patients with anaplasia.

10.3.4 Indication for Surgery for Pulmonary Metastasis

Metastases should be treated with chemotherapy and usually respond well to it. Surgery for persistent pulmonary metastasis is indicated to guide the need for radiotherapy.

10.3.5 Special Situations

Bilateral tumors and tumors with vascular extension should ideally be treated in reference centers.

10.3.5.1 Vascular Extension

Both protocols mandate neoadjuvant chemotherapy for tumor thrombus extending up to the hepatic vein or above in order to try to avoid the need for cardiopulmonary bypass and prevent complications.

Surgery for WT with intravascular extension should be performed at referral centers and in collaboration with the cardiothoracic team for patients with diaphragmatic and supradiaphragmatic extension of the thrombus. Although patients with supradiaphragmatic thrombus extension require cardiopulmonary bypass, for patients with transitional diaphragmatic level thrombus (up to the level of hepatic veins), cardiopulmonary bypass may be avoided by achieving supradiaphragmatic vena cava, hepatic vein control, and complete liver isolation; however, bypass backup should be readily available if safe control above the thrombus was not achieved. Cavotomy and thrombus resection are indicated when there is blood flow around the thrombus. On the other hand, a robust venous collateral drainage is already established whenever there is complete cava occlusion without flow; thus ligation of the contralateral vein is safe when performing cavectomy, which is the procedure of choice in this situation. Cava replacement is not physiologically needed (Fig. 10.1).

10.3.5.2 Bilateral Tumors

Both in COG and SIOP protocols, nephron-sparing resection is indicated for patients with a predisposition, such as bilateral WT, solitary kidney, or horseshoe kidney. Vascular anatomy in horseshoe kidneys can be tricky, and the surgeon should be very careful when planning the nephron-sparing procedure for such cases. Neoadjuvant chemotherapy should be used for 6–12 weeks, depending on tumor response. If there is no tumor response, surgery should be indicated, not biopsy, for it would only postpone surgery. The rational of surgery in bilateral cases is cure and renal function preservation. Some cases may need more than one surgical procedure.

Imaging cannot determine the feasibility of bilateral nephron-sparing surgery.

Open laparotomy is indicated to operate on bilateral tumors, and both kidneys can be approached in one surgical procedure or in staged procedures. Nodulectomies or heminephrectomies are indicated, depending on the anatomy and relation of the tumor with vascular structures. Manual compression on the renal hilar vessels or the parenchyma for bleeding control and gentle handling of the hilar vessels prevents vasospasm in very young patients with small blood vessels. Intraoperative ultra-

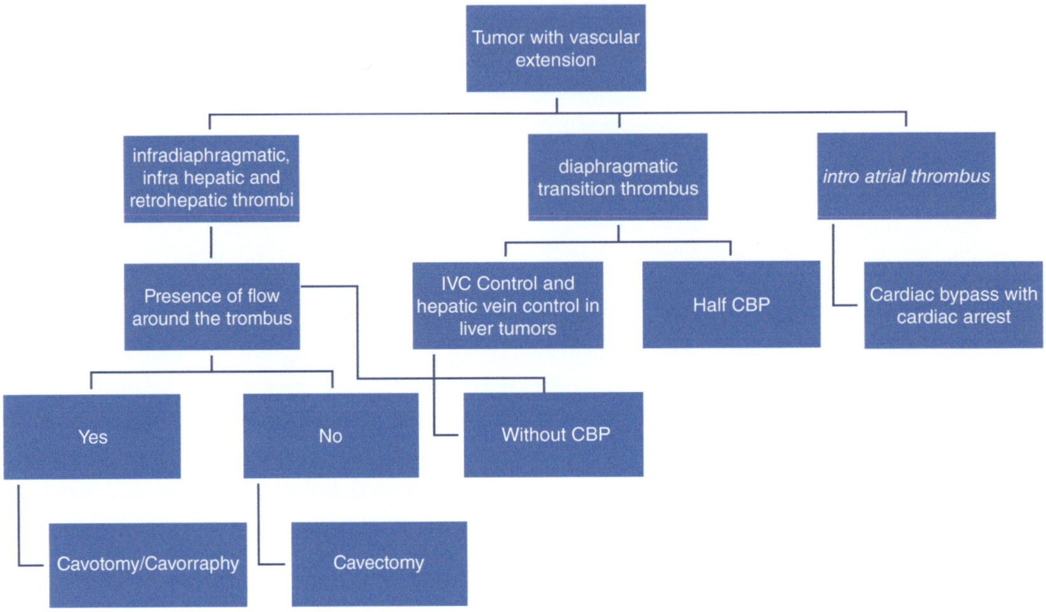

Fig. 10.1 The decision-making process for tumors with vascular extension [9]

sound can facilitate the identification of multifocal lesions and delineate the extent of each tumor if it is not clear by visual or manual inspection. This is particularly important in some cases of nephroblastomatosis, where nodules can be difficult to identify. Lymph node sampling is very important, and each kidney should be staged separately. A double J stent or perinephric drains are not routinely used but should be considered when resection involves complex collecting system reconstruction. Surface cooling is described in literature, but not usually needed, neither are bench surgery and autotransplantation techniques.

In case diffuse anaplasia is found in the context of a positive margin, completion nephrectomy is advised.

10.4 Complications

- End-stage renal failure in unilateral and bilateral WT is 0.2% and 12%, respectively, and this risk is higher in patients with predisposition syndromes, especially the Denys-Drash syndrome.
- Intussusception and adhesions are low and should be considered if the patient develops signs of obstruction.
- Significant lymphatic vessels should be ligated with suture to avoid postoperative chyle ascites [10].

10.5 Prognosis

Wilms tumor treatment is a successful example of a multidisciplinary approach, having approximately 90% survival rates in favorable histology cases.

Patients who have blastemal predominance (>65% blastema) after treatment with neoadjuvant chemotherapy have a higher rate of relapse and inferior outcomes on International Society of Pediatric Oncology (SIOP) protocols (49–52). Blastemal predominance prior to chemotherapy is not associated with poor clinical outcomes.

Diffuse anaplasia is associated with resistance to treatment and accounts for 50% of Wilms tumor deaths.

Surgeon's Checklist

1. MDT discussion.
2. Consider differential diagnoses.
3. Evaluate tumor relation to vessels and surrounding organs.
4. Evaluation of contralateral kidney at images to rule out or confirm bilateral tumors.
5. Consider the possibility of vascular extension, and if it exists, preop images should give information on thrombus level and presence/absence of blood flow around it to guide the surgical strategy.
6. Be careful not to ligate of the contralateral renal vein or superior mesenteric artery, especially in huge tumors where the anatomical landmarks are distorted.
7. Lymph node sampling is mandatory.
8. Avoiding rupture is key.
9. Surgery for persistent pulmonary metastasis is indicated to guide the need for radiotherapy.
10. Proper documentation of the procedure.

References

1. Davidoff AM. Wilms tumor. Adv Pediatr Infect Dis. 2012;59(1):247–67.
2. Khanna G, et al. Evaluation of diagnostic performance of CT for detection of tumor thrombus in children with Wilms tumor: a report from the Children's Oncology Group. Pediatr Blood Cancer. 2012;58(4):551–5.
3. Morris L, Squire R, Sznajder B, et al. Optimal neoadjuvant chemotherapy duration in Wilms tumour with intravascular thrombus: a literature review and evidence from SIOP WT 2001 trial. Pediatr Blood Cancer. 2019;66(11):e27930. https://doi.org/10.1002/pbc.27930.
4. Ribeiro RC, Schettini ST, Abib Sde C, et al. Cavectomy for the treatment of Wilms tumor with vascular extension. J Urol. 2006;176(1):279–283; discussion 283–4. https://doi.org/10.1016/S0022-5347(06)00561-1.
5. Schettini ST, da Fonseca JH, Abib SC, et al. Management of Wilms' tumor with intracardiac extension. Pediatr Surg Int. 2000;16(7):529–32. https://doi.org/10.1007/s003839900334.
6. Shamberger RC, Ritchey ML, Haase GM, et al. Intravascular extension of Wilms tumor. Ann Surg. 2001;234(1):116–21. https://doi.org/10.1097/00000658-200107000-00017.
7. Abib SCV, Chui CH, Cox S, et al. International Society of Paediatric Surgical Oncology (IPSO) surgical practice guidelines. ecancer. 2022;16:1356. https://doi.org/10.3332/ecancer.2022.1356.
8. van den Heuvel-Eibrink MM, et al. Position paper: Rationale for the treatment of Wilms tumour in the UMBRELLA SIOP-RTSG 2016 protocol. Nat Rev Urol. 2017;14(12):743–52.
9. Fanelli MCA, Guilhen JCS, Duarte AAB, et al. Management of pediatric tumors with vascular extension. Front Pediatr Sec Pediatric Surgery. 2021;9:753232. https://doi.org/10.3389/fped.2021.753232.
10. Ritchey ML, Shamberger RC, Haase G, et al. Surgical complications after primary nephrectomy for Wilms' tumor: report from the National Wilms' Tumor Study Group. J Am Coll Surg. 2001;192(1):63–68; quiz 146. https://doi.org/10.1016/S1072-7515(00)00749-3.

11 Neuroblastoma

Joshua N. Honeyman and Michael P. LaQuaglia

11.1 Introduction

Neuroblastoma is the most common extracranial solid tumor in childhood. There is a spectrum of clinical presentation that ranges from indolent disease not requiring treatment through high-risk disease requiring extensive multimodal therapy and aggressive surgical intervention. Neuroblastoma poses a therapeutic challenge requiring a multidisciplinary approach that requires specific expertise in subspecialty services, including oncology, surgery, radiology, pathology, radiation oncology, bone marrow transplantation, and others.

Internationally, the incidence of neuroblastoma ranges from 4 to 15 cases per million in children under 14 years of age [1], with one third of cases diagnosed in the first year of life and 90% of cases diagnosed within the first 5 years of life. The tumors typically arise from within the adrenal gland or along the anatomic distribution of the sympathetic nervous system.

J. N. Honeyman
Memorial Sloan Kettering Cancer Center (MSKCC), New York, NY, USA
e-mail: HoneymaJ@mskcc.org

M. P. LaQuaglia (✉)
Joseph H. Burchenal Chair in Pediatrics, Memorial Sloan Kettering Cancer Center (MSKCC), New York, NY, USA
e-mail: laquaglm@mskcc.org; delagrap@mskcc.org

11.2 Diagnosis

Presenting signs and symptoms depend on the sites of primary and metastatic disease. Most commonly, the workup is initiated when an abdominal mass is palpated. Additional findings may include distention, pain, diarrhea, fever, hypertension, anemia, bruising, and skin nodules. Periorbital disease can cause proptosis and periorbital bruising, known as "raccoon eyes." Horner's syndrome can be found with cervical and upper thoracic masses [2]. Opsoclonus/myoclonus syndrome and cerebellar ataxia are rare paraneoplastic syndromes respectively associated with rapid repeated eye movements, jerking of the extremities, and loss of balance. While patients with opsoclonus myoclonus syndrome often have favorable oncologic outcomes, the neurologic symptoms can be persistent and difficult to treat [3].

Diagnostic workup of patients with presumed neuroblastoma includes imaging, laboratory evaluation, and tumor biopsy. The differential diagnosis for neuroblastoma typically includes Wilms tumor, lymphoma, ganglioneuroma, ganglioneuroblastoma, paragangliomas, ovarian tumors, hepatoblastoma, rhabdomyosarcoma, rhabdoid tumors, desmoplastic small round cell tumor, and inflammatory myofibroblastic tumors. While many pediatric patients initially undergo screening ultrasound evaluation of abdominal pathology, cross-sectional imaging with CT or MRI is essential to characterize the extent of disease in patients with a differential diagnosis including neuroblas-

L. Krauel (ed.), *Survival Handbook in Pediatric Surgical Oncology*,
https://doi.org/10.1007/978-3-031-65890-7_11

toma. Early recognition of image-defined risk factors (IDRFs) is essential for preoperative planning prior to considering resection or biopsy. Metaiodobenzylguanidine (MIBG) scanning demonstrates avidity in the majority of neuroblastoma tumors, and it is useful both at diagnosis and in the follow-up setting [4, 5]. Positron emission tomography (PET) scans can be considered in patients who have non-MIBG-avid disease. In addition to standard screening laboratory, investigation including complete blood count, metabolic panel, hepatic panel, coagulation studies, and random urine catecholamine levels (vanillylmandelic acid/VMA, homovanillic acid/HVA) provides additional diagnostic support.

Tumor biopsy is often the first essential role of the pediatric surgeon in the care of a patient with presumed neuroblastoma. The primary goal is to safely obtain adequate tissue for the histopathologic evaluation and molecular characterization of the tumor. Depending on the stage of the tumor and the presence of IDRFs, the biopsy sample may be excisional or incisional. The surgical approach should be tailored to the patient and may include laparoscopic, open, or percutaneous techniques. Inadequate tissue volume can compromise the ability to obtain an adequate diagnosis and can lead to incorrect staging and risk stratification. At least 1 cm^3 is the minimal required volume of tissue in order to have adequate sample for histopathology, immunohistochemistry, cytogenetics, and next-generation sequencing. If a percutaneous approach is preferred, core needle size and the number of passages must be optimized to ensure the amount of tissue obtained is viable and adequate for analysis [6]. Given the vascularity of neuroblastic tumors, the risk of significant intraoperative and postoperative hemorrhage must be considered. Liberal utilization of hemostatic agents and coagulation devices is imperative.

11.3 Staging

The staging and risk stratification of neuroblastoma have evolved with better understanding of the genomic foundation of the disease. Currently, the International Neuroblastoma Risk Group Staging System (INRGSS; see Table 11.1) and the International Neuroblastoma Risk Grouping (INRG; see Table 11.2) are utilized to guide clinical decisions [7–10].

The INRGSS groups patients on preoperative extent of disease based on evaluation of imaging studies obtained at diagnosis. The staging system includes local disease without IDRFs (L1), locoregional disease with IDRFs, and two categories of metastatic disease (M and MS). There are two classic metastatic patterns that are distributed within specific age groups. Stage MS (previously Stage 4S), which occurs in children less than 18 months of age, presents with tumor spread limited to the skin, liver, and/or bone marrow, often with a favorable prognosis. In older children, metastatic disease has a poor prognosis, with metastases occurring in the cortical bone, bone marrow, lymph nodes, orbits, liver, skin, lungs, and brain.

Key to the INRGSS are IDRFs (see Table 11.1) which have been associated with increased risk of intraoperative complications, incomplete tumor resection, and worse survival. A thorough assessment and review of these risk factors will guide the surgeon through operative planning and execution.

The INRG assigns neuroblastoma patients to pretreatment risk groups based on INRG stage as well as assessment of age, histological category, grade of tumor differentiation, MYCN amplification status, presence of 11q aberration, and ploidy status. The patients are clustered into four risk levels: very low risk, low risk, intermediate risk, and high risk (Table 11.2).

Table 11.1 International Neuroblastoma Risk Group Staging System (INRGSS) and image-defined risk factors (IDRF)

International Neuroblastoma Risk Group Staging System	
Stage	*Description*
L1	Localized tumor not involving vital structures as defined by the list of image-defined risk factors and confined to one body compartment
L2	Locoregional tumor with presence of one or more image-defined risk factors
M	Distant metastatic disease (except MS)
MS	Metastatic disease in children younger than 18 months with metastases confined to skin, liver, and/or bone marrow
Image-defined risk factors (IDRF)	
Ipsilateral tumor extension within two body compartments	Neck-chest, chest-abdomen, abdomen-pelvis
Neck	Tumor encasing carotid and/or vertebral artery and/or internal jugular vein
	Tumor extending to base of skull
	Tumor compressing the trachea
Cervico-thoracic junction	Tumor encasing brachial plexus roots
	Tumor encasing subclavian vessels and/or vertebral and/or carotid artery
	Tumor compressing the trachea
Thorax	Tumor encasing the aorta and/or major branches
	Tumor compressing the trachea and/or principal bronchi
	Lower mediastinal tumor, infiltrating the costo-vertebral junction between T9 and T12
Thoraco-abdominal	Tumor encasing the aorta and/or vena cava
Abdomen/pelvis	Tumor infiltrating the porta hepatis and/or the hepatoduodenal ligament
	Tumor encasing branches of the superior mesenteric artery at the mesenteric root
	Tumor encasing the origin of the coeliac axis, and/or of the superior mesenteric artery
	Tumor invading one or both renal pedicles
	Tumor encasing the aorta and/or vena cava
	Tumor encasing the iliac vessels
	Pelvic tumor crossing the sciatic notch
Intraspinal tumor extension whatever the location provided that	More than one third of the spinal canal in the axial plane is invaded and/or the perimedullary leptomeningeal spaces are not visible and/or the spinal cord signal is abnormal
Infiltration of adjacent organs/structures	Pericardium, diaphragm, kidney, liver, duodeno-pancreatic block, and mesentery
Conditions to be recorded, but not considered IDRFs	Multifocal primary tumors
	Pleural effusion, with or without malignant cells
	Ascites, with or without malignant cells

Table 11.2 International neuroblastoma risk group

INRG stage	Age (months)	Histology	Grade	MYCN	11q	Ploidy		Pretreatment risk group
L1/L2		GN maturing/intermixed					A	Very low
L1		Any		Non Amp			B	Very low
				Amp			K	High
L2	<18	Any, except GN maturing or GNB intermixed		Non Amp	No		D	Low
					Yes		G	Intermediate
	≥18	Ganglioneuroblastoma nodular; neuroblastoma	Differentiating	Non Amp	No		E	Low
					Yes		H	Intermediate
			Poorly differentiated or undifferentiated	Non Amp				
				Amp			N	High
M	<18			Non Amp		Hyperploid	F	Low
	<12			Non Amp		Diploid	I	Intermediate
	12 to ≤18			Non Amp		Diploid	J	Intermediate
	<18			Amp			O	High
	≥18						P	High
MS	<18			Non Amp	No		C	Very low
					Yes		Q	High
				Amp			R	High

11.4 Treatment

For low-risk patients, treatment is either expectant observation or surgical resection. Chemotherapy is reserved for symptomatic patients.

Intermediate-risk patients typically have a tumor biopsy followed by neoadjuvant chemotherapy including doxorubicin, cyclophosphamide, a platinum drug, and etoposide. Most patients will proceed to surgical resection although select patients may be observed.

High-risk patients require aggressive multimodal therapy including multiple cycles of high-dose combination chemotherapy, surgery, radiation therapy, tandem autologous stem cell transplant, isotretinoin, granulocyte-macrophage colony-stimulating factor (GM-CSF), and immunotherapy, such as chimeric GD2-targeted antibody therapies (including dinutuximab and naxitamab). The role of MIBG-therapy in combination with the backbone of upfront therapy is currently being investigated in clinical trials for this high-risk population.

Major improvements have been seen in the outcomes of patients with neuroblastoma over the past 35 years, due to the application of multimodal therapy in high-risk disease, including tandem autologous transplants and complete surgical resection after completion of initial cycles of chemotherapy. In addition, immunotherapy with chimeric GD2-targeted antibodies has led to increased rates of cure and duration of disease response. Current published a 5-year overall survival for revised Children's Oncology Group (COG) risk groups are 97.9% for low-risk, 95.8% for intermediate-risk, and 62.5% for high-risk patients [9]. Despite these reported outcomes, there continues to be an unmet need for high-risk patients, with a 40% relapse rate despite intensive multidisciplinary interventions, leading to a pattern of relapsing disease that ultimately results in poor survival outcomes.

11.5 Surgical Approaches

Initial procedural interventions for neuroblastoma include biopsy, assessment of the bone marrow, and placement of central venous access. Aggressive attempts at upfront resection, particularly in the presence of IDRFs, are associated with increased risk of complications in the absence of demonstrable improvement in outcome.

11.5.1 Low-Risk Disease

For low-risk disease, treatment may consist of surgical resection or observation. Primary resection of the tumor is acceptable in properly selected patients, particularly in the absence of IDRFs. Depending on the anatomic location and the preference of the surgeon, laparoscopic and open approaches may be appropriate. Chemotherapy is reserved for select symptomatic patients. The COG biology study ANBL00B1 demonstrated a 97.9% 5-year overall survival in this risk group [9].

11.5.2 MS Disease

MS disease with favorable biology is managed with supported care given high rates of spontaneous regression and salvage. Patients with MYCN amplification or 11q aberrations are classified and managed as per the high-risk neuroblastoma treatment algorithms. Rare complications of low-risk disease include hepatomegaly, respiratory insufficiency, coagulopathy, and multisystem organ failure. Symptomatic management of these complications is personalized and may include operative interventions such as decompressive laparotomy to relieve abdominal compartment syndrome.

11.5.3 Intermediate-Risk Disease

The optimal surgical management of intermediate-risk neuroblastoma has not been definitively resolved. Outside of infants with upfront resectable disease, these patients benefit from chemotherapy as part of their treatment plan, and neoadjuvant therapy can result in a reduction in tumor volume that facilitates eventual surgical management. The goal of surgical resection in these patients is to safely resect as much disease as possible. Given response rates to chemotherapy, the risk of heroic attempts at gross total resection increases the risk of postoperative complications without impacting outcomes. Results from COG study ANBL0531 showed that treatment of intermediate-risk disease with surgery, chemotherapy, or a combination of the modalities led to favorable survival rates, with an overall survival of 94.9% [11]. Resection status (defined as >90% resection vs. <90% resection—including biopsy only) was not associated with a difference in overall survival.

11.5.4 High-Risk Disease

The surgical management of high-risk disease neuroblastoma occurs in the setting of patients receiving intensive multimodal therapy that includes neoadjuvant chemotherapy, tandem myeloablative adjuvant chemotherapy with stem cell transplant, radiation therapy, and immunotherapy. Given the presence of IDRFs in these patients, surgical resection typically requires extensive vascular dissection, neural foraminal involvement, extensive bulky adenopathy, and potential involvement of adjacent organs.

Regarding the necessary extent of surgical resection, studies from the COG and SIOPEN have demonstrated a consistent correlation between more extensive resection and overall survival. COG study A3973 reported improved overall survival in patients who underwent a >90% resection based on surgeon report [12]. The HR-NBL1/SIOPEN Study found that complete macroscopic excision was associated with improved overall survival and local control.

11.5.5 Site-Specific Considerations

11.5.5.1 Cervical

Most cervical neuroblastomas occur in infants. A transverse collar incision provides adequate exposure with access to vascular structures proximally and distally. Exposure can be facilitated by vertically extending the collar incision along the sternocleidomastoid or division of the sternocleidomastoid and strap muscles to expose underlying structures. In the setting of grossly positive lymph nodes, a completion modified neck dissection is typically indicated.

11.5.5.2 Cervicothoracic

Tumors extending through the thoracic inlet can occupy space within both the superior mediastinum and neck. For unilateral lesions, a trap-door thoracotomy comprising an anterior thoracotomy at the fifth interspace with mini sternotomy and collar incision provides excellent exposure. For tumors extending across the midline, a clamshell thoracotomy can also be considered.

11.5.5.3 Thoracic

Twenty percent of neuroblastoma arise in the posterior mediastinum. Standard assessment of preoperative risk is essential to ensure a safe procedure with good oncologic outcome. Pulmonary function, tracheal compression, and locally advanced tumor all must be assessed preoperatively. Lung isolation should be considered via double-lumen endotracheal tube or endobronchial device, and low-flow insufflation can be useful during thoracoscopy.

Posterior lateral thoracotomy via a muscle-sparing approach provides access to the posterior mediastinum and paraspinal tumors. In select cases, sternotomy provides access to the anterior mediastinum and great vessels. As for cervicothoracic lesions, clamshell and hemi-clamshell incisions allow vascular control and visualization of the brachial plexus.

Minimally invasive approaches utilizing both thoracoscopic and robotic techniques to thoracic disease have become common in cases of low-risk tumors and favorable anatomy. In carefully selected patients, oncologic outcomes have been shown to be equivalent to open approaches.

11.5.5.4 Abdomen

The adrenal glands and retroperitoneum are the most common sites for neuroblastoma, and there are many surgical approaches to abdominal neuroblastoma. A vertical midline laparotomy provides access to the abdominal structures and is particularly useful for mid-abdominal lesions extending into the pelvis. Access to upper abdominal vascular structures and retro-hepatic space can be limited without extensions to the incision. Transverse upper abdominal, subcostal, and chevron incisions along with their modifications also provide broad access to the upper abdomen.

For tumors above the renal vessels and those involving the celiac axis, a thoracoabdominal incision provides excellent exposure to the upper abdomen, the chest, the diaphragm, and the inferior mediastinum, and it has been shown to be well tolerated in the pediatric population. It provides early access to obtain proximal and distal control of major vascular structures, allowing for proximal control in the abdomen or the chest.

In select patients with L1 disease, minimally invasive approaches to abdominal neuroblastoma have been associated with decreased blood loss, pain, and length of hospital stay. However, there has been no effect on operative complications or survival.

11.5.5.5 Pelvic

Neuroblastoma arising in the pelvis originates along the sympathetic chain or organ of Zuckerkandl. Bowel and bladder dysfunction due to lumbosacral involvement is a common risk factor. Exposure of the deep pelvis is typically best achieved via midline laparotomy.

11.6 Pitfalls and Special Situation

Preservation of vascular structures and solid organs should be prioritized during resection of neuroblastoma. Attempts to avoid nephrectomy are important given risk of posttreatment renal failure and the need for intensive postoperative therapy that may require dose limitation in the setting of a single remaining kidney.

Involvement of peripheral nerve structures and neural foramina requires preoperative preparation including consideration of neurosurgical consultation, arranging intraoperative neural monitoring, and appropriate preoperative counseling of patients and families. Dumbbell tumors are paraspinal tumors that extend through neural foramina into the spinal canal. In cases of acute or evolving neurological symptoms, urgent neurosurgical consultation is necessary with consideration of chemotherapy, radiation, or laminectomy. Minimal disease entering the foramina can often be gently dissected and then transected to avoid risk of cerebrospinal fluid (CSF) leak and nerve root injury. Tumors extending along the inferior posterior mediastinum carry additional risk of spinal devascularization via the artery of Adamkiewicz.

Major hemorrhage is a considerable risk of vascular dissection associated with high-risk neuroblastoma resection. The infiltrative growth pattern of neuroblastoma leads to growth encasing major vascular structures. Dissection along a subadventitial plane can free the tumor off of these structures. Tumor can be bivalved to aid in exposure. Excellent vascular surgical technique and early proximal and distal vascular control are essential. Utilization of hemostatic adjuncts including electrothermal devices and topical hemostatic agents.

Placement of hemoclips in the region of the resection can help to guide subsequent radiation therapy.

Chyle leaks are a common complication of neuroblastoma surgery, necessitating meticulous clipping or tying of lymphatics during the course of the lymphatic dissection. If encountered in the postoperative period, conservative management is typically sufficient. Total parenteral nutrition (TPN) and/or medium chain triglycerides (MCT) formulas can lead to early resolution. Re-exploration with ligation of lymphatics or the thoracic duct is rarely indicated. Percutaneous approaches have also been described.

Potential late complications from intensive neuroblastoma therapy are numerous and include neurological, endocrine, musculoskeletal, and cardiopulmonary systems. The risk of secondary malignancies is increased in neuroblastoma survivors, particularly in high-risk patients. Long-term follow-up clinics provide excellent supportive care for neuroblastoma survivors and can provide both counseling and coordination of care for their long-term health concerns.

Surgeon's Checklist

Preoperative

1. Appropriate staging, workup, and risk stratification are essential to guide management.
2. Assembling multidisciplinary team including pediatric surgery, pediatric oncology, pediatric radiology, pediatric pathology, and neurosurgery.
3. Adequate pretreatment assessment of oncologic and operative risk.
4. Review of cross-sectional imaging focusing on staging and the identification of image-defined risk factors.
5. Consider consultation with subspecialty services (e.g., neurosurgery) early to aid with operative planning for complex resections.
6. Goal of surgery is to achieve gross total resection where possible while preserving end organ function.

Intraoperative

1. General
   (a) Attempt upfront resection for localized (L1) tumors.
   (b) Initial biopsy L2 and metastatic tumors.
   (c) Definitive resection for L2 disease following neoadjuvant chemotherapy.
   (d) Clear documentation of resection, site of disease essential.
2. Biopsy
   (a) Adequate tissue sampling for molecular biology studies.
   (b) Surgical approach to biopsy based on the patient's clinical status and tumor. Anatomy—laparoscopic, open, and percutaneous all viable.
   (c) Excellent hemostasis essential; prepare necessary adjuncts in advance.
   (d) Consultation with pathology to ensure adequate biopsy prior to leaving operating room.
3. Very Low Risk and Low Risk
   (a) Observation versus complete primary tumor resection when safe and feasible.
4. Intermediate Risk
   (a) Resection of as much tumor as safely possible, at least 50%.
5. High Risk
   (a) Optimizing incision for access to major vascular structures.
   (b) Early proximal distal control of major vascular structures.
   (c) Preservation of major vascular structures and organs.
   (d) Dissection of tumor off vessels utilizing a subadventitial plan.
   (e) Utilization of adjunct tools to aid in hemostasis (i.e., argon beam coagulator, bipolar forceps).
   (f) Resection of all gross disease when possible. Prognosis is associated with completeness of resection.
   (g) No formal lymph node dissection necessary for staging or therapeutic indications. But obviously involved regional lymph nodes are removed.
   (h) R0 resection is rarely feasible and the goal is R1 resection.

Postoperative

1. Multidisciplinary approach to pain control. Consider epidural analgesia.
2. Monitoring for complications based on surgery-specific risk factors—major hemorrhage, renal failure, neurologic complications (e.g., Horner's, foot drop, paralysis), chyle leaks, and ventilator-dependent respiratory failure.

References

1. Okawa S, Saika K. International variations in neuroblastoma incidence in children and adolescents. Jpn J Clin Oncol. 2022;52(6):656–8.
2. Graef S, Irwin MS, Wan MJ. Incidence and prognostic role of the ocular manifestations of neuroblastoma in children. Am J Ophthalmol. 2020;213:145–52.
3. Patel A, Fischer C, Lin YC, Basu EM, Kushner BH, De Braganca K, et al. Treatment and revaccination of children with paraneoplastic opsoclonus-myoclonus-ataxia syndrome and neuroblastoma: The Memorial Sloan Kettering experience. Pediatr Blood Cancer. 2020;67(8):e28319.

4. Kushner BH, Kramer K, Modak S, Cheung NK. Sensitivity of surveillance studies for detecting asymptomatic and unsuspected relapse of high-risk neuroblastoma. J Clin Oncol. 2009;27(7):1041–6.
5. Bleeker G, Tytgat GA, Adam JA, Caron HN, Kremer LC, Hooft L, et al. 123I-MIBG scintigraphy and 18F-FDG-PET imaging for diagnosing neuroblastoma. Cochrane Database Syst Rev. 2015;2015(9):CD009263.
6. Overman RE, Kartal TT, Cunningham AJ, Fialkowski EA, Naik-Mathuria BJ, Vasudevan SA, et al. Optimization of percutaneous biopsy for diagnosis and pretreatment risk assessment of neuroblastoma. Pediatr Blood Cancer. 2020;67(5):e28153.
7. Cohn SL, Pearson AD, London WB, Monclair T, Ambros PF, Brodeur GM, et al. The International Neuroblastoma Risk Group (INRG) classification system: an INRG Task Force report. J Clin Oncol. 2009;27(2):289–97.
8. Brisse HJ, McCarville MB, Granata C, Krug KB, Wootton-Gorges SL, Kanegawa K, et al. Guidelines for imaging and staging of neuroblastic tumors: consensus report from the International Neuroblastoma Risk Group Project. Radiology. 2011;261(1):243–57.
9. Irwin MS, Naranjo A, Zhang FF, Cohn SL, London WB, Gastier-Foster JM, et al. Revised neuroblastoma risk classification system: a report from the Children's Oncology Group. J Clin Oncol. 2021;39(29):3229–41.
10. Monclair T, Brodeur GM, Ambros PF, Brisse HJ, Cecchetto G, Holmes K, et al. The International Neuroblastoma Risk Group (INRG) staging system: an INRG Task Force report. J Clin Oncol. 2009;27(2):298–303.
11. Twist CJ, Schmidt ML, Naranjo A, London WB, Tenney SC, Marachelian A, et al. Maintaining outstanding outcomes using response- and biology-based therapy for intermediate-risk neuroblastoma: a report from the Children's Oncology Group Study ANBL0531. J Clin Oncol. 2019;37(34):3243–55.
12. von Allmen D, Davidoff AM, London WB, Van Ryn C, Haas-Kogan DA, Kreissman SG, et al. Impact of extent of resection on local control and survival in patients from the COG A3973 study with high-risk neuroblastoma. J Clin Oncol. 2017;35(2):208–16.

Liver Tumors in Children

12

Ines Moraleda Gudayol and Michael Berger

12.1 Diagnosis

The diagnosis of malignant hepatic tumors in children is often due to the presence of a **large palpable mass** in the upper abdomen. Initially, children with these tumors generally exhibit good clinical condition. However, as the disease progresses, symptoms such as abdominal pain, weight loss, loss of appetite, anemia, and vomiting may arise. Ascites is uncommon and not a typical symptom of hepatic tumors in children. Liver function is usually maintained, although prominent and diffuse lung metastases can occasionally cause respiratory insufficiency. The most significant risk factors for hepatoblastoma include extreme premature birth, the Wiedemann-Beckwith syndrome, other hemihypertrophies, and familial polyposis coli (FAP) [1, 2].

Primary liver tumors are a significant occurrence in childhood, ranking as the third most common abdominal tumor after neuroblastomas and kidney tumors. In Central Europe, the incidence of these tumors ranges from 0.5 to 2 cases per 1 million individuals, constituting approximately 0.3–2% of all pediatric tumors [3]. The most prevalent type of primary liver tumor in children is hepatoblastoma. Liver tumors can be broadly categorized into two groups.

I. M. Gudayol
Department of Pediatric Surgery, Essen University Hospital, Essen, Germany

Department of Pediatric Surgery, University of Sydney, Sydney, NSW, Australia
e-mail: ines.moraleda@uk-essen.de

M. Berger (✉)
Department of Pediatric Surgery, Essen University Hospital, Essen, Germany
e-mail: michael.berger@uk-essen.de

12.1.1 Benign Liver Tumors

- *Hepatic hemangioma (HH)*: HH is the most prevalent benign hepatic tumor in children. It is typically diagnosed in early infancy (before 6 months of age) and rarely causes symptoms. In instances where symptoms do arise, successful treatment with propranolol is often feasible. In very rare cases, aggressive behavior may be observed in these tumors, necessitating surgical resection. The underlying reasons for this minuscule subset of aggressive hemangiomas remain unknown, although recent research has identified an over-activation of the hedgehog-signaling pathway in specimens of such tumors.
- *Focal nodular hyperplasia (FNH)*: FNH is more likely to occur in older children and adolescents. It can also occur in circumstances that provoke poor portal flow to the liver, like in cases of congenital portosystemic shunts.
- *Hepatocellular adenomas (HAs)*: HAs are typically seen in older children.

L. Krauel (ed.), *Survival Handbook in Pediatric Surgical Oncology*,
https://doi.org/10.1007/978-3-031-65890-7_12

- *Mesenchymal hamartoma*: Mesenchymal hamartoma is a rare benign liver tumor primarily affecting infants and young children. It typically presents as a large, multicystic mass within the liver, often diagnosed during prenatal ultrasound or in the early postnatal period. Although typically benign, mesenchymal hamartomas can cause significant morbidity due to mass effect, compression of adjacent structures, or rupture. Surgical resection is the mainstay of treatment, with excellent long-term outcomes following complete excision. However, careful monitoring and follow-up are essential due to the potential for recurrence. Further research is needed to better understand the pathogenesis and optimal management strategies for this uncommon pediatric liver tumor.

12.1.2 Malignant Liver Tumors

These tumors exhibit distinct characteristics and are commonly associated with specific age groups.

- *Hepatocellular (HB)*: Is an embryonal tumor and usually manifests before or around the age of 3 years.
- *Hepatocellular carcinoma (HCC)*: HCC primarily affects older children and adolescents (5–16 years), with rare occurrences in young children.
- *Hepatocellular neoplasm-not otherwise specified (HCN-NOS)*: One specific consideration is the transitional liver cell tumor (TLCT), now often referred to as HCN-NOS (NOS = not otherwise specified). This tumor exhibits histological features of both hepatoblastoma and HCC and is sometimes characterized by the presence of a telomerase reverse transcriptase promoter (TERP) mutation at the molecular level. Although these tumors may exhibit clear signs of HCC on histology, they do show signs of b-catenin/Wnt-signaling, a clear feature of hepatoblastoma, and behave more aggressively like hepatoblastomas. TLCTs tend to occur in otherwise healthy livers of children during their early school age, accompanied by elevated levels of alpha-fetoprotein (AFP), albeit not as high as typical hepatoblastoma. Unlike true HCC, TLCTs often show a remarkable response to chemotherapy. In cases where complete surgical removal through upfront resection is uncertain, preoperative chemotherapy is recommended. It is essential to bear in mind that post-chemotherapy biopsies of TLCTs may falsely indicate the presence of HCC due to the selective elimination of more responsive hepatoblastoma cells. Consequently, these children should be treated as having aggressive hepatoblastoma.
- *Undifferentiated embryonic sarcoma of the liver*: This tumor typically presents in children aged 5–10 and is usually AFP-negative.
- *Rhabdomyosarcoma of the bile ducts*: This tumor usually presents with jaundice due to bile duct obstruction and is usually AFP-negative.
- *Rhabdoid tumor of the liver*: Rhabdoid tumors of the liver have a dismal prognosis and typically young children around the age of 1 year. This tumor is characteristically negative for AFP. See Table 12.1 below, for age distribution of liver tumors.

Table 12.1 Age distribution of liver tumors [2, 8]

	Infants and toddlers	School age and adolescents
Malignant	Hepatoblastoma Rhabdomyosarcoma	Hepatocellular carcinoma Undifferentiated embryonal sarcoma
Benign	Hemangioma Mesenchymal hamartoma	Adenoma Focal nodular hyperplasia

12.2 Diagnostic Tests

In addition to routine blood count, C-reactive protein (CRP), and liver enzymes, the tumor markers **AFP, β-HCG, ferritin, LDH,** and **CEA** should be investigated. Hepatoblastomas usually have very high AFP levels; however, low AFP levels do not exclude the diagnosis of hepatoblastoma but rather indicate a poor prognosis. For imaging, in addition to ultrasound either a **CT** scan or an **MRI** is mandatory for the pre-treatment extension (PRETEXT) group of the tumors [4]. A **chest CT scan** should also be performed to rule out lung metastases.

12.3 Staging

The staging of malignant primary liver tumors in childhood has been extensively studied, and various classification systems have been developed. One of the widely accepted staging systems is the **PRETEXT** ("pre-treatment extension") system, introduced by the *Société Internationale d'Oncologie Pédiatrique*—Epithelial Liver Tumor Study Group (SIOPEL). This system relies on pre-therapeutic imaging and is independent of surgical or therapeutic procedures. The PRETEXT is expressed as a number that assesses the extent of the tumor in the four surgical sectors of the liver and incorporates letter-defined risk factors. The PRETEXT system has demonstrated significant prognostic relevance and is widely used in the international scientific literature pertaining to hepatoblastoma.

Another staging system used in some studies, particularly in North America until recently, is the grouping system developed by the Children's Oncology Group (COG) [5]. This system is based on the assessment of tumor resectability, which is a subjective measure dependent on the surgeon's expertise. Consequently, it is considered less reliable compared to the PRETEXT grouping system [6].

More recently, the Children's Hepatic Tumors International Collaboration (CHIC), a worldwide coalition dedicated to the study of hepatoblastomas, has developed a new risk stratification system. This system incorporates data from over 1600 children treated over a period of 25 years. It utilizes several factors, including the PRETEXT classification, the initial alpha-fetoprotein (AFP) value at diagnosis, the presence of metastases, vascular invasion, and the age of the child. Based on these factors, the CHIC risk stratification system defines four risk levels: very low, low, intermediate, and high. Currently, this risk stratification system is being employed in the ongoing Pediatric Hepatic International Tumor Trial (PHITT) study [1].

All things considered, the current liver tumor staging is as follows:

- **PRETEXT group** (expressed with a number I to IV): describes the number of adjoining tumor-free liver sections. It determines the number of contiguous sections that would have to be resected to completely remove the tumor [6, 7] (see Image 12.1).
- **PRETEXT annotation factors** (expressed with a letter): involvement of the hepatic veins and/or the inferior vena cava (V), portal venous involvement (P), involvement of the

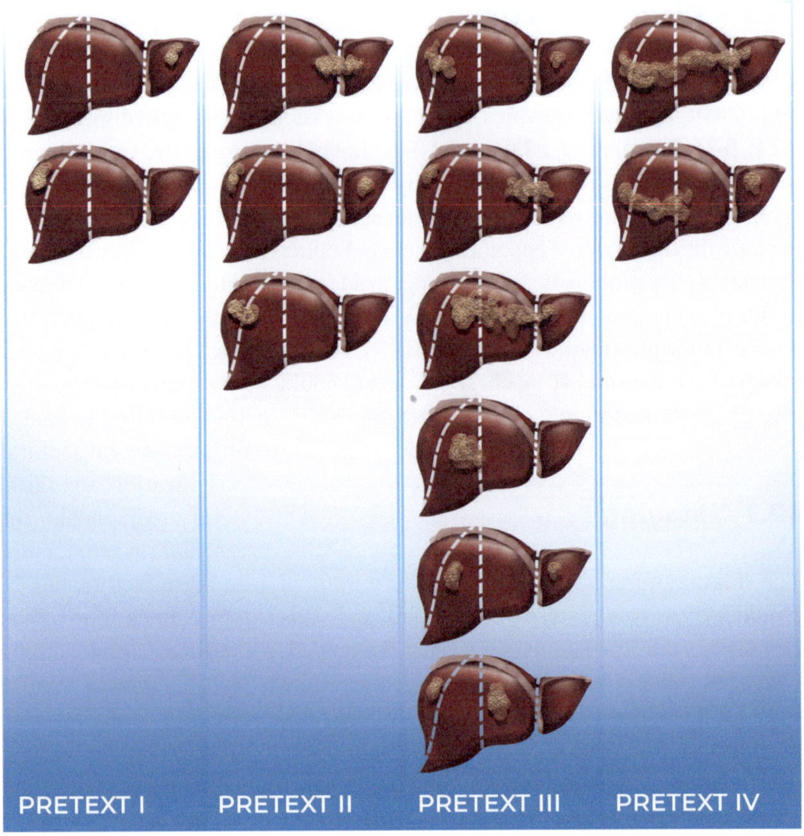

Image 12.1 PRETEXT classification. (Extracted from Ng and Mogul [8])

caudate lobe (C), presence of extrahepatic intra-abdominal tumor (E), tumor focality (F), distant metastases (M), lymph node metastases (N), and tumor rupture (R) [5, 8].

12.4 Treatment

Hepatoblastomas, like other embryonic tumors in children, exhibit favorable responses to chemotherapy. Several commonly used agents have shown good efficacy in treating these tumors, including cisplatin, carboplatin, doxorubicin, ifosfamide, etoposide, vincristine, and 5-fluorouracil. It is worth noting that after repeated administration of chemotherapy, hepatoblastoma cells often develop significant resistance to cytostatic effects. This is also true for other malignant liver tumors in childhood.

Currently, the PHITT study, a global multicenter research study, is underway to investigate optimal treatment strategies for children diagnosed with hepatoblastoma or hepatocellular carcinoma (HCC) in children. This multinational study aims to evaluate various chemotherapeutic regimens and establish guidelines for deciding between surgical resection and primary liver transplantation. The trial is registered under the identification number NCT03017326.

12.5 Surgical Approaches

12.5.1 Biopsy

Historically, hepatic tumors that showed the typical signs of hepatoblastoma (large tumor, typical characteristics on imaging, young age, high AFP) were treated without biopsy. According to the latest SIOPEL trial (PHITT), this approach is now obsolete, and **all tumors should get a**

biopsy before starting chemotherapy. [9] The only exception to this understanding is a PRETEXT I or II tumor with more than 1 cm margin to large vessels on imaging that can be removed with simple hemihepatectomy. Only these tumors may have an upfront resection without prior biopsy. The usual work-up of a liver tumor typically does not entail extensive molecular genetic studies. Therefore, the US-guided core biopsy, either percutaneous or laparoscopic-assisted, of the tumor is the method of choice. If the tumor is poorly accessible percutaneously or very well perfused, an open biopsy may be indicated. Fine-needle biopsy with cytology is insufficient in most cases and not a standard of care.

12.5.2 Surgical Resection

Surgical resection plays a pivotal role in the therapeutic approach to hepatoblastoma. Complete resection of the tumor is essential for achieving a cure in cases of hepatoblastoma. Therefore, the prognosis for non-resectable hepatoblastoma has been historically unfavorable. However, the introduction of primary liver transplantation as a means of achieving complete surgical resection has brought about a revolutionary change in hepatoblastoma therapy over the past decade. This approach has provided new opportunities for treatment and improved outcomes for patients.

Major liver resection (removal of three or more adjacent segments) is a safe surgery when performed in a tertiary liver center. It should be based on the Glissonian technique (see Image 12.2), to identify the ligation point of the vascular pedicles to ensure good perfusion of the remaining liver. Intraoperative ultrasound can be useful to guide resection, to identify either vessels or tumor margins.

The parenchymal transection of the liver should be performed by ligature or Kelly clamp crushing technique, to minimize bleeding.

Nonanatomical resections should be avoided for all malignant liver tumors because they have been shown to have a higher rate of complications and a higher recurrence rate.

There are currently no clear guidelines for the role of laparoscopic approaches. At all times, complete surgical resection with negative margins is paramount, as malignant liver tumors are curable only if complete surgical eradication is achieved. Isolated studies have also been published for laparoscopic partial hepatectomies and left lateral segmentectomies for malignant liver tumors, and results have been adequate. These techniques should only be performed after a care-

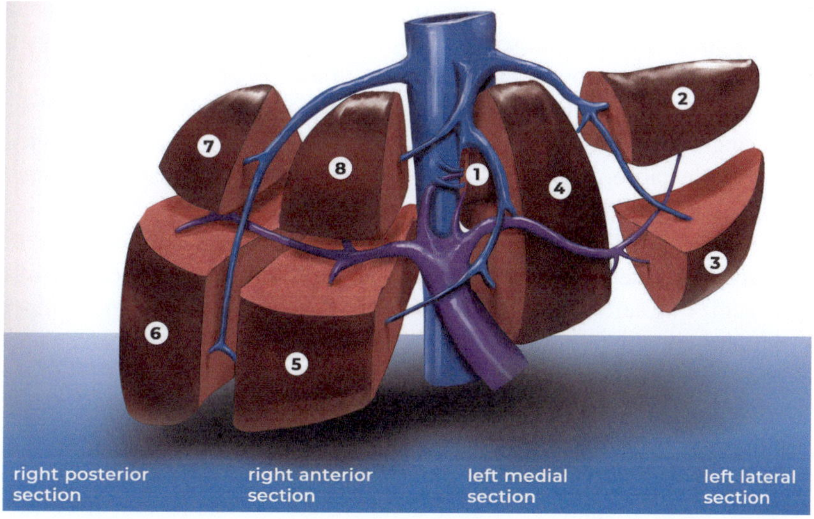

Image 12.2 Surgical anatomy of the liver. (Modified from Roebuck et al. [6])

ful patient selection and multidisciplinary committee evaluation.

The resection of lung metastases in case of residual disease following chemotherapy should be actively considered, as it has been demonstrated in a number of studies that it improves outcome.

12.6 Liver Transplantation

To this day, it is not entirely clear which constellation of liver tumors requires resection versus liver transplantation. As a hallmark, it needs to be re-emphasized that malignant liver tumors are curable only with complete resection of the tumor. Whether this is achieved via resection of liver transplantation is irrelevant. Based on previously published research, the following scenarios in hepatoblastoma may indicate the need for a liver transplant [10, 11]:

- Multifocal tumors, particularly multifocal PRETEXT IV tumors with tumor presence in all four liver sections at the time of diagnosis. This of all constellations is the most clear-cut indication for liver transplantation over resection.
- Unifocal PRETEXT IV tumors, even if they "downstage" to a posttreatment extent of disease (POST-TEXT) III through neoadjuvant chemotherapy but still require trisegmentectomy for conventional resection.
- PRETEXT III tumors with involvement of the vena cava or all three major hepatic veins, raising concerns about achieving adequate tumor clearance.
- PRETEXT III tumors with proximity to the portal venous bifurcation or both major branches of the portal vein, posing challenges in achieving sufficient tumor clearance.
- Intrahepatic relapse or residual tumor following a previous attempted resection or re-resection, often referred to as "rescue transplant."

In the case of hepatoblastoma in children, the presence of extrahepatic tumors does not necessarily rule out the possibility of a liver transplant. If all metastases can be effectively eliminated through surgery or chemotherapy, liver transplantation remains a viable option. It is important to note that primary liver transplant for hepatoblastoma has shown excellent results, with survival rates exceeding 85%. Salvage liver transplant, performed after unsuccessful resection attempts, has traditionally been thought to have poorer outcomes, with survival rates around 30%. However, more recent international data suggest that high success rates can be achieved even in this patient population if candidates are selected carefully. Careful patient selection entails selecting children that have recurrent disease confined only to the liver that show a solid AFP-response during application of rescue chemotherapy and who, after hepatectomy, have anatomical prerequisites and options for a technically sound implantation of the graft (e.g., open portal vein for inflow reconstruction). Therefore, if complete surgical resection by traditional means appears doubtful initially, every effort should be made to prioritize primary liver transplant as a means of achieving successful surgical resection.

12.7 Pitfalls

- Inadequate tissue sampling can lead to unclear diagnosis. A fine-needle aspiration biopsy is not accepted for a valid histopathological diagnosis. Always try to obtain tissue with a biopsy [12].
- Relying on AFP serology: serum AFP levels can be physiologically raised until 6 months of age. Also, some low-differentiated tumor subtypes may have normal serum AFP.
- Not sharing your cases in multicenter study groups. Because of the rarity of these tumors, it is of utmost importance that the knowledge is shared between the work groups.

Surgeon's Checklist

1. Hepatoblastoma is not only the most common malignant liver tumor during childhood but also the most common liver tumor overall.

Therefore, any new or growing lesion in the liver of a child needs thorough investigation.
2. AFP is an excellent tumor marker for diagnosing and following treatment response of hepatoblastoma. However, remember that AFP-negative lesions may still be malignant and often are because these tumors can be either AFP-negative hepatoblastomas, rhabdoid tumors of the livers or embryonal sarcomas of the liver. All the mentioned tumors usually have a rather poor prognosis compared to the typical APF-high hepatoblastoma.
3. When considering resection versus transplant, it is advisable to comply to current guidelines described by the SIOPEL.
4. If complete resection seems doubtful or needs extraordinary measures like ex vivo reconstruction or use of the heart-lung machine, don't do it. The data is against you.
5. Despite the many pitfalls that most certainly do exist in pediatric liver transplant, in experienced centers, pediatric liver transplant is the standard therapy with excellent long-term results.
6. A tumor that has not become resectable after the risk-stratified preoperative chemotherapy has been given will remain unresectable. Don't delay liver transplantation by giving more chemotherapy in an ill-advised attempt to try to make it resectable. The tumor cells will have developed an insensitivity against the chemotherapy, and it will not work.
7. Recurrent hepatoblastoma has a very poor prognosis, and no current guidelines exist for its treatment. Some success has been seen when complete surgical clearance of tumor burden can be achieved, especially in localized disease.
8. Rescue liver transplant in recurrent hepatoblastoma confined to the liver has traditionally been believed to have very a bad outcome. However, newer international data suggest that it is a successful treatment option if patients are selected carefully.

References

1. Kastenberg ZJ, Meyers RL. Liver tumors. In: Mattei P, editor. Fundamentals of pediatric surgery. 1. Switzerland: Springer Cham; 2022. p. 1033–46.
2. Davenport M. Liver tumors. In: Sinha CK, Davenport M, editors. Handbook of pediatric surgery. 2. Switzerland: Springer Cham; 2022. p. 381–9.
3. Von Schweinitz D. Hepatoblastoma: recent developments in research and treatment. Semin Pediatr Surg. 2012;21:21–30.
4. Yikilmaz A, George M, Lee EY. Pediatric hepatobiliary neoplasms: an overview and update. Radiol Clin N Am. 2017;55:741–66.
5. Honeyman JN, La Quaglia MP. Malignant liver tumors. Semin Pediatr Surg. 2012;21(3):245–54.
6. Roebuck DJ, et al. 2005 PRETEXT: a revised staging system for primary malignant liver tumours of childhood developed by the SIOPEL group. Pediatr Radiol. 2007;37:123–32.
7. Towbin AJ, Meyers RL, Woodley H, et al. 2017 PRETEXT: radiologic staging system for primary hepatic malignancies of childhood revised for the Paediatric Hepatic International Tumour Trial (PHITT). Pediatr Radiol. 2018;48:536–54.
8. Ng K, Mogul DB. Pediatric liver tumors. Clin Liver Dis. 2018;22(4):753–72.
9. Ranganathan S, Lopez-Terrada D, Alaggio R. Hepatoblastoma and pediatric hepatocellular carcinoma: an update. Pediatr Dev Pathol. 2020;23(2):79–95.
10. Berger M. Transplantation in children. In: Lacher M, St. Peter SD, Zani A, editors. Pearls and tricks in pediatric surgery. 1. Switzerland: Springer Cham; 2020. p. 477–83.
11. Boster JM, Superina R, et al. Predictors of survival following liver transplantation for pediatric hepatoblastoma and hepatocellular carcinoma: experience from the Society of Pediatric Liver Transplantation (SPLIT). Am J Transplant. 2022;22:1396–408.
12. Morgan Auld F, Sergi CM. Surgical pathology diagnostic pitfalls of hepatoblastoma. Int J Surg Pathol. 2022;30(5):480–91.

13 Paediatric Lymphoma: The Surgeon's Role

Sharon Cox

13.1 Introduction

Lymphomas are a heterogeneous group of malignancies stemming from the reticuloendothelial system, typically developing in lymph nodes or primary lymphoid organs, but they can present as solid tumours almost anywhere in the body. Lymphoma is the third most common paediatric cancer, totalling between 10 and 15% of childhood malignancies. Males account for over 60% of cases, and Caucasians are more likely to be affected. Children under age 14 are most likely to have fast-growing, aggressive non-Hodgkin's lymphoma (NHL), while older children and teens are more likely to have Hodgkin's lymphoma (HL).

13.2 Types of Lymphoma

The surgeon should have a basic understanding of the common types of lymphoma, their incidence and presentation to allow for informed surgical management decisions. NHL accounts for approximately 60% of childhood lymphomas.

S. Cox (✉)
Health Sciences Faculty, Division of Paediatric Surgery, University of Cape Town, Cape Town, South Africa

Division of Paediatric Surgery, Red Cross War Memorial Children's Hospital, Cape Town, South Africa
e-mail: sharon.cox@uct.ac.za

13.2.1 Non-Hodgkin's Lymphoma

- Burkitt's lymphoma (40% of childhood NHL) is a fast-growing B-cell lymphoma that commonly presents as a large abdominal mass and spreads quickly. Endemic forms often appear as a jaw mass, or with loose teeth.
- Diffuse large B-cell lymphoma (10–20% of childhood NHL) can arise anywhere including nodes and the bone marrow, thyroid, brain gastrointestinal tract, liver, spleen and testes with a rare subtype presenting as a large mass in the mediastinum.
- Anaplastic large cell lymphoma is a heterogeneous group of B and predominantly T-cell lineage lymphomas that often present in the nodes and spread to the skin, bones, liver lung and soft tissues and account for just over 10% of childhood NHL.
- Lymphoblastic lymphoma (approximately 20% of childhood NHL) is normally T cell in origin and commonly affects teens and males and often presents in lymph nodes or the thymus.

13.2.2 Hodgkin's Lymphoma [1]

- Classic HL accounts for 80% of childhood HL and is further classified into four main types:
  - Nodular-sclerosing Hodgkin's lymphoma commonly presents in adolescents. A medi-

L. Krauel (ed.), *Survival Handbook in Pediatric Surgical Oncology*,
https://doi.org/10.1007/978-3-031-65890-7_13

astinal mass is a common presentation in this subtype.
  - Mixed cellularity Hodgkin's lymphoma is often associated with Epstein-Barr virus, and generally presents with an enlarged neck node in children younger than 10.
  - Lymphocyte-rich and lymphocyte-depleted subtypes are rare in children.
- Nodular lymphocyte predominant Hodgkin's lymphoma that accounts for 10% of paediatric HL generally occurs in children younger than 10 and presents as a cervical or axillary nodal mass, usually without any other symptoms.

13.3 Patient Presentation

Along with the heterogeneity of lymphoma and the multiple sites it may involve comes a wide variation in the presenting symptoms and signs. Patients can present with nonspecific symptoms, enlarged lymph nodes or an abdominal mass or various surgical diagnoses such as intussusception or appendicitis which may be the first presentation with diagnosis confirmed on subsequent histology.

Nonspecific symptoms include:

- Persistent fatigue.
- Weight loss.
- Fever and night sweats.
- Easy bruising.
- Recurrent infections.

For nodal masses, the following are concerning signs that should prompt biopsy [2]:

- Fast-growing masses.
- Persistent nodes beyond 2–3 weeks of duration, unresponsive to antibiotics.
- Multiple levels of lymphadenopathy.
- Supraclavicular location.
- Hard and fixed nodes.

Features of thoracic lymphoma may include:

- Supraclavicular nodes.
- Shortness of breath or orthopnoea.

Abdominal lymphoma presentations include [3, 4]:

- Abdominal pain.
- Organomegaly.
- Features of bowel obstruction or peritonitis from intestinal perforation.
- Gastrointestinal bleeding.
- Urinary tract obstruction.

Surgeons thus need to be aware of the varied and multiple possible presentations as the possibility of lymphoma influences surgical management decisions.

13.4 Patient Assessment

As with any patient presenting with a suspicious mass, full blood workup including blood counts, clotting profile, liver and renal functions, as well as relevant tumour markers—specifically lactate dehydrogenase (LDH) when lymphoma is suspected—should be performed.

Imaging studies relevant to the site and nature of the presentation may include radiographs, ultrasound or cross-sectional imaging.

Of particular note in patients with mediastinal or thoracic disease is the need to assess the impact of the mass on the airway by chest X-rays or CT, as general anaesthetic and recumbent position may lead to life-threatening airway obstruction due to compression by the mass [2].

Imaging of large abdominal masses is needed to assess the relationship of the mass to the abdominal organs, which are often involved, displaced by or enclosed within the tumour mass. This is especially relevant when the mass involves the bowel and mesentery, as biopsy of the bowel wall can lead to complications such as bowel perforation and enterocutaneous fistula in these patients.

13.5 The Role of the Surgeon

Where lymphoma is concerned, it is important that the surgeon works as part of a well-functioning multidisciplinary team (MDT). The role of the surgeon within this team is predominantly that of obtaining sufficient tissue for precise diagnosis by means of various histological techniques. Other roles include the management of common childhood surgical presentations that are later proven to be an initial presentation of lymphoma, management of surgical complications of advanced disease or due to chemotherapy, as well as supportive procedures such as the insertion of central venous access devices (CVADs).

Patients may be referred to the surgeon for:

- Biopsy of a suspicious node or mass.
- Prior to diagnosis of lymphoma for surgery for other childhood surgical conditions, or acute abdomen.
- Management of complications of chemotherapy including bowel perforation.
- Insertion of a central venous access device (CVAD) for chemotherapy, or haemodialysis line for tumour lysis syndrome.
- Biopsy of a residual mass after chemotherapy.

13.6 Tumour Biopsy

Tumour biopsy may be:

- Excisional biopsy: this preserves the nodal architecture.
- Incisional biopsy under vision (minimally invasive or open approach).
- Image-guided core biopsy (ultrasound or CT).

Complete resection of the mass is normally not needed and could be destructive if attempted. A sample of sufficient tissue for appropriate histological analysis including genetic and molecular phenotyping should be acquired. Fine-needle aspiration biopsy is generally not sufficient for the number of histological processes required for accurate diagnosis and subtyping [2, 5].

To minimize surgical morbidity, the most superficial and easily accessible mass should be biopsied first. For deeper lesions, it is advisable to choose the least invasive method of biopsy that is safe and will obtain sufficient representative tissue. Thoracoscopy and laparoscopy are preferred if feasible, but if deemed unsafe or difficult, thoracotomy or laparotomy can be considered [5]. Destructive surgery involving excision of large, complex masses should be avoided.

It is best to discuss with the pathologist how they would like to receive the specimen. Fresh specimens are preferred, as opposed to those sent in preservatives such as formalin. The surgeon should also oversee labelling, handling and transfer of the specimens.

In patients undergoing biopsy, it is advisable to determine the need for further procedures under the same anaesthetic to increase efficiency and decrease further anaesthetics. This is especially relevant when frozen section during the procedure will determine the nature of the mass and thus inform further decisions. Preoperative consent should be taken for all potential procedures, such as insertion of CVAD, bone marrow biopsy, lumbar puncture or thoracocentesis.

13.6.1 Considerations in Lymph Node Biopsy

Patients presenting with enlarged nodes and symptoms suspicious of non-benign lesions will need a node biopsy. Supraclavicular nodes should always be biopsied as almost a quarter of these will show malignancy.

The technique and site should be individualized to the patient's condition. Taking the accessibility of the node into account, the largest and most firm node should be biopsied. Should there be multilevel disease, for best yields, supraclavicular, cervical and axillary followed by inguinal biopsy is the site order of choice [6]. It is important to remember that in areas with endemic TB or high HIV prevalence, patients may have concurrent pathologies. In the case of a small superficial node, an excisional biopsy is preferred for full histological assessment and disease classification [2, 5].

13.6.2 Biopsy Considerations in Thoracic Lesions

Orthopnoea is a predictor of respiratory collapse at induction of anaesthesia. Either a 50% reduction in predicted expiratory flow rate or the predicted tracheal diameter is a contraindication to general anaesthesia [7]. In these situations, the surgeon is advised to search for a representative peripheral node to biopsy or pleural fluid to tap under local anaesthetic in a more upright position. If there are no other sites and biopsy of a large mediastinal mass is required, the anaesthetist should be well prepared, adjust sedation, use specific intubation and difficult airway equipment and position the patient in the most suitable manner.

13.6.3 Biopsy Considerations in Abdominal Disease

Burkitt's lymphoma often presents as a rapidly enlarging abdominal mass with or without malignant ascites [4]. It often involves the mesenteric nodes (more commonly in high-income countries) but can present in or around any abdominal organ.

It may be difficult to reliably demonstrate and define the bowel on imaging as the bowel wall may be infiltrated (more common in low-income countries). Inadvertent biopsy of the bowel wall may lead to perforation and resultant fistulization; thus open biopsy under direct vision is preferred to image-guided biopsy in these situations.

For gonadal disease, incision as opposed to excision biopsy should be performed.

13.7 Acute Surgical Presentations

Acute presentations leading to emergency surgery are also common. Intussusception with lymphoma as a lead point may occur in Burkitt's lymphoma and mature B-cell NHL more commonly and less frequently in post-transplant lymphoproliferative disease. Concerning factors such as a lead point on ultrasound, irreducibility, recurrence and a non-ileo-colic site will generally lead to surgical exploration at which time it may be possible for a full excisional biopsy by resection and anastomosis of the involved bowel [3].

Abdominal lymphoma may also mimic acute appendicitis. Disease may be confined to the appendix, or, more commonly, involve the bowel mesentery, retroperitoneal and intra-abdominal areas. In this situation, incisional biopsy is warranted, taking care not to damage the bowel wall or retroperitoneal structures.

In emergent presentations of bowel obstruction or perforation resulting from a complex intra-abdominal tumour mass, the best approach is control of bowel contents via a proximal diverting stoma and tumour biopsy at the same setting to stabilize the patient and confirm the diagnosis. Resection and bowel anastomosis in this setting has a high risk of breakdown, sepsis and even death—especially in the face of chemotherapy in the postoperative period.

Less commonly, patients may present with an isolated, small mass involving a short segment of bowel and mesentery. In this instance resection of a short segment and anastomosis can be safely performed, it is preferable to do so as this reduces chemotherapy—which should be delayed a few days to allow for healing of the anastomosis.

Gastrointestinal bleeding should be dealt with as per institutional protocols that would include full blood workup and then endoscopy and biopsy of any suspicious lesions.

13.8 Surgical Complications of Lymphoma Treatment

Medical therapy for lymphoma is highly effective. Large masses shrink over days to weeks after commencement of chemotherapy, and this is particularly marked in Burkitt's lymphoma. The rapid regress of extensive bowel wall involvement may lead to bowel perforation, intra-abdominal collections and sepsis. Patient management needs to be individualized; the focus is to clear intra-abdominal collections to manage sepsis and divert the effluent. Resection and anastomosis of involved areas should be avoided in these patients as they are generally neutropenic and in a poor physiological state. In this situation, stoma creation is preferred.

In the longer term, infrequent bowel obstruction due to strictures in areas of previous mucositis may develop. Generally, at this stage the patient is out of the acute phase and has a physiologically improved condition; thus resection and anastomosis may be performed.

13.9 Venous Access Requirements

For the most part, lymphoma is a medically managed condition, necessitating the need for central venous access devices for chemotherapy administration. Important considerations when inserting these devices revolve around issues related to sepsis and clotting—especially in those with bone marrow involvement. Prior to theatre, full blood workup is required, and any anomalies should be corrected. If possible, the device should be inserted at the time of biopsy under the same anaesthetic to avoid multiple visits to theatre. Insertion should be delayed in the face of sepsis or haemodynamic instability. Prophylactic antibiotics on insertion are advised. The surgeon should follow their existing protocols for line insertion [2].

Haemodialysis lines may be needed in patients with Burkitt's lymphoma and/or massive tumour burden. Ordinarily this line is a temporary 'push-in' line and may be inserted in the intensive care unit, on the ward or in the radiology suite by interventional radiologists. The surgeon may be involved in this procedure or may need to facilitate it under the same anaesthetic as other surgical procedures.

All CVAD and lines should be inserted after consultation within the multidisciplinary team managing the patient.

13.10 Surgical Role in Residual Masses

While residual disease is not common due to the efficacy of therapy, re-imaging at the time of clinical remission or end of chemotherapy protocol may detect a residual mass. Neither initial tumour size nor the size of the residual mass is a predictor of residual disease. Conventional imaging techniques have a high sensitivity in mass detection but a low sensitivity in determining the difference between disease and necrosis or fibrosis in paediatric B-cell NHL [8].

In NHL, 18F-fluoro-2-deoxy-d-glucose positron emission tomography (FDG-PET) may be used to help differentiate the nature of the residual mass. Persistent abnormal [18F] FDG uptake after first-line chemotherapy in NHL is highly, but not completely predictive of residual or recurrent disease, so biopsy confirmation should be performed if feasible [9]. In patients with non-avid residual masses, a watch-and-wait approach can be applied.

In HL tumour masses contain large amounts of collagen and fibrous stroma which may result in residual masses of non-viable tissue after chemotherapy [1]. FDG-PET/CT is the current standard for assessment in HL [1]. Patients with non-avid residual masses do not have worse outcomes than those without a residual mass [10]. It is thus prudent to clinically monitor these patients. For masses taking up FDG-PET where the nature of the mass is in doubt, the easily accessible residual mass should be biopsied by the least invasive manor, be that image-guided, via minimally invasive or open techniques.

A difficult situation arises when a small residual mass of unknown nature is present in an area that would require extensive surgery to access. In these circumstances management should be individualized in the context of the patient, imaging and pathology. Ongoing observation and follow-up may be appropriate to avoid invasive approaches—and as with surgery relating to all residual masses, decisions on any surgical procedure would need to be made within the multidisciplinary team.

Surgeon's Checklist

1. Develop a basic understanding of the types of lymphoma and their presentations to enable informed surgical decisions.
2. Be aware of the varied presentations as the possibility of lymphoma influences surgical management decisions.
3. When taking a child to theatre for a biopsy, determine further procedures such that they may be performed at the same time.
4. In the patient with multiple potential biopsy sites, biopsy the most representative and accessible lesion.
5. Obtain sufficient representative tissue in the safest and least invasive manner.
6. In abdominal disease involving the bowel, open biopsy under vision is preferred to avoid biopsy of the bowel wall.
7. Discuss exact handling and transport of the biopsy specimen with the pathologist.
8. Extensive, destructive surgery and excision of complex abdominal masses are not indicated.
9. Diversion via a stoma is preferred to resection and anastomosis, particularly in unstable patients with complex masses.
10. Should resection and anastomosis be performed in suitable situations, chemotherapy should be postponed allowing time for anastomotic healing.
11. Gonadectomy is not indicated; if the gonad is involved, it should be biopsied.
12. For residual masses after treatment, surgical management should be individualized according to available clinical, imaging and pathological information in the setting of a MDT meeting.

References

1. Kluge R, Kurch L, Georgi T, Metzger M. Current role of FDG-PET in pediatric Hodgkin's lymphoma. Semin Nucl Med. 2017;47(3):242–57.
2. de Campos Vieira Abib S, Chui CH, Cox S, Abdelhafeez AH, Fernandez-Pineda I, Elgendy A, et al. International society of paediatric surgical oncology (IPSO) surgical practice guidelines. Ecancermedicalscience. 2022;16:1356.
3. Bussell HR, Kroiss S, Tharakan SJ, Meuli M, Moehrlen U. Intussusception in children: lessons learned from intestinal lymphoma as a rare lead-point. Pediatr Surg Int. 2019;35(8):879–85.
4. Shamberger RC, Weinstein HJ. The role of surgery in abdominal Burkitt's lymphoma. J Pediatr Surg. 1992;27(2):236–40.
5. Yahanda AM. Lymphoma. In: Holzheimer RG, Mannick JA, editors. Surgical treatment evidence based and problem orientated. Munich: Zuckschwerdt; 2001.
6. Grant CN, Aldrink J, Lautz TB, Tracy ET, Rhee DS, Baertschiger RM, et al. Lymphadenopathy in children: a streamlined approach for the surgeon—a report from the APSA cancer committee. J Pediatr Surg. 2021;56(2):274–81.
7. Perger L, Lee EY, Shamberger RC. Management of children and adolescents with a critical airway due to compression by an anterior mediastinal mass. J Pediatr Surg. 2008;43(11):1990–7.
8. Cai M, Wang T, Pan C, Gao Y, Zhou M, Hu W, et al. Investigating the potential benefit of second biopsy of residual mass in pediatric mature B cell non-Hodgkin lymphoma. Pediatr Hematol Oncol. 2019;36(2):113–21.
9. Rahman HA, El Semary SF, Ahmed G, Kenaai NE, Omar W, Zaky I, Nagy N. Can FDG-PET replace biopsy for the evaluation of residual tumor in pediatric mature B-cell non-Hodgkin lymphoma? Pediatr Blood Cancer. 2020;67(9):e28310.
10. Adams HJ, Nievelstein RA, Kwee TC. Outcome of Hodgkin lymphoma patients with a posttreatment 18F-fluoro-2-deoxy-d-glucose positron emission tomography (FDG-PET)-negative residual mass: systematic review and meta-analysis. Pediatr Hematol Oncol. 2015;32(8):515–24.

Soft Tissue Sarcomas

14

Gabriela Guillén Burrieza
and Marta Martos Rodríguez

14.1 Introduction

Pediatric soft tissue sarcomas (STS) are a heterogeneous group of malignant tumors derived from primitive mesenchymal cells. They are classified into rhabdomyosarcomas (RMS) and non-rhabdomyosarcoma soft tissue sarcomas (NRSTS).

We will summarize the current management of these tumors; however, the treating surgeon must be familiar with the treatment protocol used in his/her center, as recommendations in diagnostic workup, surgical guidelines, and treatment plans differ among collaborative groups. Otherwise, consultation with a reference team is highly advised. The most widespread used protocols are those from the Children's Oncology Group (COG) and the European Paediatric Soft Tissue Sarcoma Study Group (EpSSG).

Rhabdomyosarcoma is the most common STS in children (55–60%). It accounts for approximately 3.5% of cancer in children between 0 and 14 years of age (one third of cases appear in children under 5 years of age), being the third most frequent extracranial solid tumor. Incidence in adolescents is lower, representing 2% of all cancers in patients between 15 and 19 years of age. There is a higher prevalence in males (1.5:1). The most frequent locations are the head and neck (35–50%), genitourinary tract (25%), and limbs (20%). Most cases are sporadic, but around 5% are associated with various tumor predisposition syndromes (Li-Fraumeni, DICER1, neurofibromatosis type 1, and Beckwith-Wiedemann syndrome, among others).

NRSTS comprise several malignant neoplasms of presumed mesenchymal origin that differ on clinical features (from locally aggressive to highly malignant), age distribution, and response to treatment. There are more than 50 different histotypes, and some of them are more prevalent in adults. These malignancies show a very low incidence.

14.2 Diagnosis

Usually, STS clinical presentation is in the form of a painless, growing tumor appearing in any part of the body. Symptoms may vary according to their anatomic location. Among RMS, 15–25% of patients have metastasis at diagnosis, the most frequent location being the lungs, followed by the bone marrow, bone, and lymph nodes. Systemic symptoms (fever, weight loss, pancytopenia) are rare and are usually indicative of disseminated disease.

G. Guillén Burrieza (✉) · M. Martos Rodríguez
Pediatric Surgical Oncology Unit, Pediatric Surgery Department, Hospital Universitari Vall d'Hebron, Barcelona, Spain
e-mail: gabriela.guillen@vallhebron.cat; marta.martosrodriguez@vallhebron.cat

L. Krauel (ed.), *Survival Handbook in Pediatric Surgical Oncology*,
https://doi.org/10.1007/978-3-031-65890-7_14

An ultrasound is usually the initial examination. Rhabdomyosarcomas will appear as a hypoechoic, heterogeneous, and highly vascularized mass; NRSTS can show different features. MRI is the gold-standard image modality for local staging, and it must include the entire anatomical region (e.g., for extremities, the entire limb) as well as the proximal lymph node basins. A CT scan might be a better option only in some locations (e.g., skull base) [1]. Lung metastases are assessed with a pulmonary CT scan. A whole-body PET/CT scan at diagnosis is essential for staging and follow-up [2]. PET/CT is especially useful for lymph node evaluation, with high sensitivity and specificity, although it does not replace lymph node biopsy. For intermediate-risk and high-risk RMS and in certain NRSTS, bone marrow aspirate and biopsy are needed, and lumbar puncture will be indicated in parameningeal tumors.

Pathology and molecular studies will give the definitive diagnosis; the surgeon or the radiologist performing the biopsy must ensure to provide enough tissue. A centralized pathology review is recommended, since the diagnosis may be challenging.

RMS is a mesenchymal tumor, similar in morphology and genomics to skeletal muscle cells. It's a small round cell tumor, and immunohistochemistry is positive for muscle proteins such as muscle-specific actin, desmin, vimentin, myosin, and myoglobin. There are three main types in children and adolescents [3]:

- Embryonal (eRMS): eRMS is the most frequent subtype (60–70%). eRMS is driven by several oncogenic mutations (*RAS*, *TP53*). This subtype is more common in younger children and has generally a more favorable prognosis; however, eRMS with *MYOD1*^{L122R} mutations associate a poor outcome.
- Alveolar (aRMS): aRMS accounts for 25% of RMS and can develop in children and adolescents. It appears more frequently in the limbs. They show characteristic fusion genes (PAX3-FOXO1 and PAX7-FOXO1) that lead to dedifferentiation and proliferation of myogenic cells and harbor a worse prognosis.
- Spindle cell: It is extremely rare (3–10%). This subtype is characterized by the presence of spindle cells with some degree of sclerosis. It develops mostly in the head and neck region, and has a poor prognosis.

Regarding NRSTS, there are three main categories: synovial sarcomas, "adult-type" sarcomas, and "other histotypes." These are summarized in Table 14.1. Molecular characterization is essential for diagnosis.

Synovial sarcoma is the most common pediatric NRSTS. It occurs most often in patients older than 10 years and can develop in any location, with the limbs being the most frequently affected region. It's a high-grade sarcoma, with a characteristic translocation t(X;18)(p11.2;q11.2) and subsequent *SYT::SSX* fusions.

"Adult-type" soft tissue sarcomas are typical of adulthood. The most common subtype is the malignant peripheral nerve sheath tumor (MPNST) that occurs mainly in patients with neurofibromatosis type 1.

The "other histotypes" are a heterogeneous group of tumors that develop typically in children and adolescents, with their own differential characteristics [4].

A biopsy will be the first surgical procedure in all cases, except for very small, localized lesions, in which a complete resection with negative margins is possible without loss of function or great morbidity. Image-guided core needle biopsy (at least four to eight cylinders, 16-14G) is the preferred method, but also surgical or endoscopic biopsies are adequate (e.g., for genitourinary tumors). Tissue must be enough for histological diagnosis, centralized review, immunohistochemistry, cytogenetics, biological studies, and preservation of frozen material. The sample must be sent fresh, preferably.

The biopsy tract has to be planned to allow the subsequent oncological resection, avoiding compromising vascular-nervous structures and respecting compartmental anatomy. Bleeding must be prevented, to avoid overstaging tumors. The use of drains is not recommended, and if necessary, they will be placed in the same direction as the incision and as close as possible to it, so that the drain tract can be resected en bloc at definitive surgery.

Current protocols recommend surgical sampling of clinically or radiologically suspicious

Table 14.1 NRSTS subtypes

Synovial sarcoma	
"Adult-type" soft tissue sarcoma	Malignant peripheral nerve sheath tumors Epithelioid sarcoma Liposarcoma Pleomorphic malignant fibrous histiocytoma/undifferentiated high-grade pleomorphic sarcoma Angiosarcoma Fibrosarcoma—Adult type Alveolar soft part sarcoma Clear cell sarcoma of tendons and aponeurosis Dermatofibrosarcoma protuberans Leiomyosarcoma Low-grade fibromyxoid sarcoma
Other histotypes	The PEComa family tumors Myoepithelial tumors Extracranial rhabdoid tumor Desmoplastic small round cell tumor Undifferentiated soft part sarcoma of the liver Undifferentiated soft part sarcoma BCL6 corepressor (BCOR) family of undifferentiated sarcomas CIC-DUX4 sarcomas Extraosseous chondrosarcoma Malignant ectomesenchymoma Fibroblastic/myofibroblastic malignancies Giant cell fibroblastoma Angiomatoid fibrous histiocytoma Plexiform fibrohistiocytic tumor Infantile fibrosarcoma and NTRK1 mesenchymal tumors Desmoid-type fibromatosis Inflammatory myofibroblastic tumors Epithelioid hemangioendothelioma

lymph nodes, at diagnosis and at relapse. Regional lymph nodes must be always biopsied in case of extremity tumors and of paratesticular tumors in patients older than 10 years. It is also advisable for tumors in the trunk, head and neck, and perianal/perineal [2]. Lymph node sampling can be performed as "berry picking" (removal of the clinically involved nodes) or preferably, through a sentinel lymph node biopsy. Lymph node involvement requires intensification of therapy due to an increased risk of relapse. Importantly, nodal disease is rare in NRSTS and limited to some histotypes, where nodal biopsy will be indicated.

14.3 Staging

14.3.1 RMS

Staging through the pretreatment TNM system (primary tumor size greater or less than 5 cm and location, lymph node involvement, and distant metastasis) and surgical pre-chemotherapy Intergroup Rhabdomyosarcoma Study (IRS) groups (Table 14.2) are the base of the different risk groups. These are complex and differ among the existing international protocols. IRS group, patient age, tumor size, PAX fusion status (and other biological markers), tumor site (favorable or unfavorable), lymph node status, and metastasis, influence the prognosis and the risk classification (Table 14.3). PAX and/or FOXO1 fusion status is one of the most important prognostic factors. Patients with localized disease who present positive fusion have a 36% 5-year disease-free survival that reaches 70% if the fusion is negative. Favorable and unfavorable anatomic sites show some differences among collaborative groups.

14.3.2 NRSTS

Staging is performed through TNM classification and IRS groups. The E*p*SSG has established the

Table 14.2 TNM and IRS groups

TNM	
T1	Tumor confined to tissue of origin
T2	Tumor beyond tissue of origin
A	≤5 cm in maximum diameter
B	>5 cm in maximum diameter
N0	No nodal involvement
NI	Nodal involvement
NX	Unknown nodal status
M0	No distant metastasis
M1	Distal metastasis
IRS	
IRS-I	Tumor completely removed, negative margins
IRS-II	(a) Microscopic residual tumor (b) Involved regional nodes (c) Both
IRS-III	Gross residual tumor after biopsy or incomplete resection
IRS-IV	Distant metastatic disease

Table 14.3 Risk groups established by the E*p*SSG, FaR-RMS protocol (2021)

Risk group	Subgroup	Site	Fusion status	IRS group	Size and age	Node stage
Low	A	Any	–	I	Both favorable	N0
Standard	B	Any	–	I	One or both unfavorable	N0
	C	Favorable	–	II,III	Any	N0
High	D	Unfavorable	–	II,III	Any	N0
	E	Any	–	II,III	Any	N1
	F	Any	+	I,II,III	Any	N0
Very high	G	Any	+	II,III	Any	N1
	H	Any	Any	IV	Any	Any

risk groups based on IRS classification, tumor size (< or >5 cm), nodal involvement, and tumor grade. For synovial sarcoma, tumor site is also a criterion. The COG risk classification considers the presence of metastases, IRS stage, size, and tumor grade.

14.4 Treatment

Multimodal treatment of pediatric sarcomas requires assessment from a multidisciplinary team and is planned in a risk-based approach. Rhabdomyosarcomas always require chemotherapy and usually a combination of surgery and/or radiotherapy. The principles of multimodal risk-adapted treatment for pediatric and adolescent NRSTS have been established very recently by the results of the COG ARST0332 and the E*p*SSG NRSTS 2005 studies [5]; treatment is adjusted to the characteristics of the different histotypes, especially their chemosensitivity, and the prognostic factors defined by previous studies. Some NRSTS have their own treatment recommendations.

14.4.1 Systemic Treatment

Neoadjuvant treatment in RMS aims to facilitate surgical approach and increase cure rates and disease-free survival. Currently, the overall 5-year survival rate in patients with localized disease is around 80% [6]. Neoadjuvant treatment consists of a combination of vincristine and actinomycin, in association with ifosfamide in E*p*SSG and cyclophosphamide in COG. Its intensity is adjusted to the risk groups.

For NRSTS, surgery is generally the keystone of treatment, if feasible. Chemotherapy can be safely omitted in tumors of intermediate malignancy and in the low-risk population. Multimodal therapy (including surgery, radiotherapy, and chemotherapy regimens, with high doses of ifosfamide and doxorubicin) is necessary when facing malignant subtypes, especially high-grade sarcomas [5]. The recent COG and E*p*SSG studies proved the ability of neoadjuvant treatment (chemotherapy, radiotherapy) to improve the results in initially unresectable cases and even facilitated delayed resection.

Synovial sarcoma and "adult-type" sarcomas are managed in a similar way, with some differences [4]. Sixty percent of pediatric synovial sarcomas are chemosensitive, but most adult-type NRSTS have little sensitivity to chemotherapy, limiting the role of systemic treatment, that is generally indicated in the case of unresectable tumors or in high-grade tumors after local treatment.

The "other subtypes" of NRSTS include a wide variety of locally aggressive (inflammatory myofibroblastic tumor, desmoid fibromatosis, infantile fibrosarcoma) and highly malignant tumors typical from children and adolescents (desmoplastic small round cell tumor (DSRCT), malignant rhabdoid tumor, undifferentiated embryonal sarcoma of the liver) with specific treatment guidelines for each of them, including some targeted therapies.

14.4.2 Local Treatment

Local control of the disease, through surgical resection and/or radiotherapy, is a fundamental part of multimodal treatment in most sarcoma patients. The selection of one modality over another or the combination of both (surgery and radiotherapy) needs to be discussed and adjusted to the patient's age, staging, histological subtype, tumor biology, tumor location, response to neoadjuvant treatment, and the experience of the treating team.

14.4.2.1 Surgery

The biopsy tract, if possible, should be included en bloc with the surgical resection. The different anatomic locations will require specific approaches [7], and the surgeon needs to develop a precise surgical plan that must include the reconstructive procedures. For some anatomic locations, like parameningeal tumors, surgery will be generally avoided, favoring radiotherapy. For other locations where severe long-term sequelae can be expected, like prostatic or perineal tumors, brachytherapy combined with a limited surgical resection (or no surgery at all) seems to be the optimal local treatment and, if possible, must be offered to the patients [8].

The quality of surgical resection is classified as follows and must appear on the surgical report as it will influence the radiotherapy planning and the intensity of the cytotoxic treatment:

- R0 (microscopically complete resection): en bloc resection including the tumor, its pseudocapsule, and a rim of healthy tissue. It is highly conditioned by the tumor's size and location and patient's age.
- R1 (microscopically incomplete resection): microscopic presence of tumor in the surgical margins, with no evidence of macroscopic disease. R1 can be the best option when dealing with major blood vessels, epineurium, or periosteum.
- "Contamination" is defined as an accidental rupture of the pseudocapsule with dissemination to the surgical field. Adjuvant radiotherapy will be generally necessary.
- R2 (macroscopically incomplete resection): macroscopic presence of tumor after resection.

The surgical specimens must be oriented and marked for pathology exams, and surgical titanium clips need to be placed at the margins of the tumor bed (cranial, caudal, lateral, and medial) and on any area of residual tumor. Intraoperative frozen sections might be necessary to confirm negative margins.

RMS

There are some possible scenarios for surgical resection, as for NRSTS:

Primary/upfront resection: It is the resection performed at diagnosis, and should only be carried out if an R0 can be guaranteed without mutilation or risk of severe complications and in cases with no nodal or metastatic disease. This is only feasible in some selected cases (tumors smaller than 3 cm, superficial, and most paratesticular). Mutilating procedures should never be considered at first surgery.

Pretreatment re-excision: Wide (non-mutilating) resection in patients with microscopic residual disease after primary resection, to achieve R0 resection. It must include the scar tissue and surrounding areas and should be performed before starting other therapies and as close as possible to the first surgery, with the aim of not delaying adjuvant chemotherapy.

Delayed primary excision: Definitive surgical resection that is performed after induction chemotherapy is the most common situation for most cases. Surgery should only be performed if an R0/R1 resection is considered possible, as debulking procedures are generally not recommended. If the response to chemotherapy has been complete (no macroscopic tumor in cross-sectional imaging), surgery is usually not indicated.

Mutilating resections may be indicated if chemotherapy and radiotherapy have not achieved local control, or if it is considered that the toxicity of radiotherapy is unacceptable (i.e., in children under 12 months of age).

NRSTS

In general, surgical principles for RMS will suit NRSTS but with some exceptions. Definitions for positive or negative surgical margins in NRSTS are different for North American and European groups [9] and for low-intermediate-grade tumors versus high-grade tumors. As a rule, the current consensus is that a minimum of 1 mm can be considered as an R0, but a 5 mm margin of surrounding healthy tissue should be the ideal goal when possible.

However, indications for surgical treatment differ among histotypes and clinical context. While for some tumors, a wait-and-see approach will be indicated (i.e., desmoid tumors), for other histologies existing targeted therapies will help to limit or even avoid aggressive surgical treatment (i.e., infantile fibrosarcoma and NTRK inhibitors, inflammatory myofibroblastic tumors, and anaplastic lymphoma kinase (ALK) inhibitors). Some NRSTS, such as synovial sarcoma, will show a significative response to neoadjuvant chemotherapy, but others will require an aggressive surgical treatment [4]. For some patients, preoperative radiotherapy can be the best option, aiming to reduce toxicity in healthy tissues and to facilitate a gross resection.

Some tumors deserve a separate comment, regarding special surgical techniques. Desmoplastic small round cell tumor (DSRCT) is a highly aggressive sarcoma, with very poor survival, that most commonly develops in the peritoneal cavity. The degree of surgical resection (R0 or R1) seems to be relevant for survival in most series, especially in localized cases. Intensive cytotoxic treatment, with complete cytoreductive surgery (CRS) combined or not with hyperthermic intraperitoneal chemotherapy (HIPEC), followed by radiotherapy, is considered by many authors as the best approach.

Dermatofibrosarcoma protuberans is a slow-growing NRSTS from the dermis, with a great tendency to local recurrence due to its infiltrative growth pattern. The best treatment is achieved by wide local excision, including microsurgical methods such as the Mohs micrographic surgery, a commonly used technique in dermatosurgery.

14.4.2.2 Radiotherapy

Radiotherapy is used for local control in patients with microscopic or macroscopic residual disease after surgical or chemotherapy treatment and for some anatomic locations (e.g., skull base). New techniques such as intensity-modulated radiation (IMRT) or proton radiotherapy can reduce the impact of this therapy in the long term, significantly reducing the dose received by the organs that are close to the tumor. Each case must be individualized and evaluated by a multidisciplinary committee.

It's indicated in around 85% of RMS patients, being necessary in almost all cases of standard, high, and very high risk tumors. The radiotherapy field should include both the primary tumor and the pathological lymph nodes.

In NRSTS, radiotherapy is usually indicated for local control after incomplete resections, as adjuvant treatment after resection of large tumors, and in some cases (mostly in COG protocols) as neoadjuvant treatment.

When radiotherapy affects the pelvic area, fertility preservation by gonadal transposition or cryopreservation should be considered.

14.5 Decision-Making

Due to their complexity and rarity, pediatric and adolescent sarcoma patients need to be treated within international protocols, by experienced multidisciplinary teams in specialized centers, and their inclusion in clinical trials is of utmost importance.

14.6 Pitfalls

1. Never perform a soft tissue mass resection without proper preoperative imaging studies that help characterize the lesion. An unplanned non-oncological resection can compromise the patient's outcome.
2. At initial biopsy, plan properly the incision or the biopsy tract, avoid bleeding and tumor rupture, and do not use drains if possible.
3. Make sure lymph nodes are sampled according to protocols. Untreated pathological nodes affect local relapse and survival.
4. Surgery should only be performed if an R0/R1 resection is considered possible. Mutilating surgeries should never be considered as first-line treatment, and reconstructive procedures need to be planned. Debulking is not recommended.
5. Avoid mutilating procedures at first surgery, although these might be necessary in some scenarios, such as local relapse or to avoid deleterious effects of radiation therapy in small children.
6. Follow oncology principles, perform en bloc surgical resection with a sufficient rim of healthy tissue, and avoid the exposure of the tumor capsule and tumor rupture. If this happens, reflect it on the report and wash abundantly the surgical field.
7. Plan the necessary reconstructive procedures, considering all the factors (the need of local radiotherapy, the continuation of the cytotoxic treatment, etc.).
8. Put the patient first: Referring the sarcoma patients to expert multidisciplinary teams is always the best option.

Surgeon's Checklist

1. When faced with a soft tissue mass, consider the possibility of a diagnosis of sarcoma and act accordingly.
2. At diagnosis, the mass should be characterized by imaging tests (being MRI the gold standard), and these should be performed appropriately, including regional lymphatic drainage areas. Chest CT and whole-body PET-CT will complete initial imaging staging.
3. In general, biopsy should be the first surgical procedure, except in the rare cases where non-mutilating surgical resection with free margins is feasible and only if there is no lymph node involvement or distant disease.
4. Percutaneous core needle biopsies are recommended (16 or 14 G needle). The access for the biopsy must respect compartmental anatomy to allow a safe oncological resection. It must provide enough tissue and should be sent fresh.
5. Lymph nodes with a pathological appearance at diagnosis and at relapse should be biopsied, if feasible. If no pathologic lymph nodes are found at imaging exams, the surgeon must know the recommendations of each protocol regarding the performance of lymph node biopsies (with or without sentinel lymph node biopsy (SLNB) techniques).
6. FOXO1 fusion status is one of the most important prognostic factors, regardless of histological group.
7. Plan the surgical resection and the reconstructive procedure.
8. The tumor bed and/or remains have to be marked with surgical titanium clips. When adjuvant radiotherapy is necessary, the field should include both the primary tumor and the pathological nodes if present.

9. The specimen needs to be oriented and marked with sutures. It's essential to keep feedback between the surgeon and the pathologist.
10. Organ-preserving techniques, such as brachytherapy, are the first treatment option for certain anatomic locations.

References

1. van Ewijk R, Schoot RA, Sparber-Sauer M, Ter Horst SAJ, Jehanno N, Borgwardt L, de Keizer B, Merks JHM, de Luca A, McHugh K, von Kalle T, Schäfer JF, van Rijn RR, Cooperative Weichteilsarkom Studiengruppe Imaging Group, the European Society of Paediatric Radiology Oncology Task Force and the European Paediatric Soft Tissue Sarcoma Study Group Imaging Committee. European guideline for imaging in paediatric and adolescent rhabdomyosarcoma—joint statement by the European Paediatric Soft Tissue Sarcoma Study Group, the Cooperative Weichteilsarkom Studiengruppe and the Oncology Task Force of the European Society of Paediatric Radiology. Pediatr Radiol. 2021;51(10):1940–51. https://doi.org/10.1007/s00247-021-05081-0. Epub 2021 Jun 17. PMID: 34137936; PMCID: PMC8426307
2. Rogers TN, Dasgupta R. Management of rhabdomyosarcoma in pediatric patients. Surg Oncol Clin N Am. 2021;30(2):339–53. https://doi.org/10.1016/j.soc.2020.11.003. Epub 2021 Jan 27
3. Skapek SX, Ferrari A, Gupta AA, Lupo PJ, Butler E, Shipley J, Barr FG, Hawkins DS. Rhabdomyosarcoma. Nat Rev Dis Primers. 2019;5(1):1. https://doi.org/10.1038/s41572-018-0051-2. PMID: 30617281; PMCID: PMC7456566
4. Ferrari A, Brennan B, Casanova M, Corradini N, Berlanga P, Schoot RA, Ramirez-Villar GL, Safwat A, Guillen Burrieza G, Dall'Igna P, Alaggio R, Lyngsie Hjalgrim L, Gatz SA, Orbach D, van Noesel MM. Pediatric non-rhabdomyosarcoma soft tissue sarcomas: standard of care and treatment recommendations from the European paediatric soft tissue sarcoma study group (EpSSG). Cancer Manag Res. 2022;14:2885–902. https://doi.org/10.2147/CMAR.S368381. PMID: 36176694; PMCID: PMC9514781
5. Ferrari A, Orbach D, Sparber-Sauer M, Walterhouse DO, Pajtler KW, Meyer WH, Spunt SL, Weiss AR. The treatment approach to pediatric non-rhabdomyosarcoma soft tissue sarcomas: a critical review from the INternational Soft Tissue SaRcoma ConsorTium. Eur J Cancer. 2022;169:10–9. https://doi.org/10.1016/j.ejca.2022.03.028. Epub 2022 Apr 28
6. Bisogno G, Minard-Colin V, Zanetti I, Ferrari A, Gallego S, Dávila Fajardo R, Mandeville H, Kelsey A, Alaggio R, Orbach D, Terwisscha van Scheltinga S, Guillén Burrieza G, Ben-Arush M, Glosli H, Mudry P, Ferman S, Devalck C, Defachelles AS, Merks JHM, Jenney M. Nonmetastatic rhabdomyosarcoma in children and adolescents: overall results of the European pediatric soft tissue sarcoma study group RMS2005 study. J Clin Oncol. 2023;41(13):2342–9. https://doi.org/10.1200/JCO.22.02093. Epub 2023 Feb 27
7. Terwisscha van Scheltinga S, Rogers T, Smeulders N, deCorti F, Guerin F, Craigie R, Burrieza GG, Smeele L, Hol M, van Rijn R, Fuchs J, Seitz G, Schmidt A, Timmermann B, Tunn PU, Chargari C, Dávila Fajardo R, Slater O, Gains J, Merks H. Developments in the surgical approach to staging and resection of rhabdomyosarcoma. Cancers (Basel). 2023;15(2):449. https://doi.org/10.3390/cancers15020449. PMID: 36672397; PMCID: PMC9857078
8. Chargari C, Haie-Meder C, Espenel S, Garcia MA, Ben-Arush M, Bolle S, Borjesson A, Cesen M, Lago RC, Defachelles AS, De Moerloose B, Devalck C, Edslev P, Farinha NJ, Francotte N, Glosli H, Gouy S, Burrieza GG, Helfre S, Irtan S, Kattamis A, Lacerda A, Levy A, Hjalgrim LL, Mansuy L, Mascard E, Moalla S, Orbach D, Owens C, Philippe-Chomette P, Pizer B, Pluchart C, Renard M, Rognlien AGW, Rome A, Sarnacki S, Safwat A, Schiavetti A, Serre J, Verite C, Weid NV, Wysocki M, Valteay-Couanet D, Deutsch E, Minard-Colin V, Martelli H, Guérin F. Brachytherapy for pediatric patients at Gustave Roussy cancer campus: a model of international cooperation for highly specialized treatments. Int J Radiat Oncol Biol Phys. 2022;113(3):602–13. https://doi.org/10.1016/j.ijrobp.2022.03.003. Epub 2022 Mar 9
9. Sparber-Sauer M, Ferrari A, Spunt SL, Vokuhl C, Casey D, Lautz TB, Meyer WH, Walterhouse DO, Pajtler KW, Alaggio R, Schmidt A, Safwat A, Timmermann B, Dall'Igna P, Chen S, Weiss AR, Orbach D. The significance of margins in pediatric non-rhabdomyosarcoma soft tissue sarcomas: consensus on surgical margin definition harmonization from the INternational Soft Tissue SaRcoma ConsorTium (INSTRuCT). Cancer Med. 2023;12(10):11719–30. https://doi.org/10.1002/cam4.5671. Epub 2023 Feb 6. PMID: 36744538; PMCID: PMC10242312

15 Ovarian Tumors in Children and Adolescents

Lucas Krauel and Albert Pasten

15.1 Introduction

Ovarian tumors are a rare condition in children, accounting for 2.6–3/100.000 girls per year. Of them, up to 20–30% can be malignant, and the presentation, etiology, and prognosis are particular for this population [1]. The surgeon has an important role in the management of ovarian tumors and should take part of the multidisciplinary team that provides care to these patients. Unlike adult patients, the goal is to achieve cure while preserving gonadal function when possible [2].

It's important to remark that the first contact with this condition could occur with a broad and heterogeneous variety of specialists: a pediatrician, a general practitioner, and a gynecologist; moreover, these tumors can manifest as a surgical emergency. The pediatric surgeon is often called for the final decision: when and/or how to operate [3]. Therefore, it is crucial to have enough knowledge to lead the actions to obtain a diagnosis as soon as possible, respecting the oncological rules of safety.

15.2 Etiology

An ovarian malignancy could appear from the different cellular types that exist in the gonad. In children and adolescents, most malignant tumors are of germinal origin, comprising 70% of the total. Epithelial origin, the most common in adults, accounts approximately only 15% of cases, rising its incidence in adolescents and young adults. Finally, stromal malignant tumors are the least frequent, with 5% of incidence, and have a bimodal presentation age, 3–4 years of age, and in adolescence. Table 15.1 shows the different types of malignancy derived from these three cellular lines.

Table 15.1 Malignant ovarian diseases and their origin

Ovarian origin	Type of tumor
Germ Cells	Dysgerminoma
	Embryonic Carcinoma
	Yolk sac tumor, choriocarcinoma
	Teratoma (mature/immature)
Epithelial cells	Benign: Serous or mucinous cystadenomas
	Malignant: Serous or mucinous carcinomas
Sex cord stromal cells	Benign: Thecomas, fibromas
	Malignant: Granulosa cell tumors, Sertoli-Leydig tumors

L. Krauel · A. Pasten (✉)
Pediatric Surgical Oncology, Pediatric Surgery Department, Pediatric Cancer Center Barcelona (PCCB), SJD Barcelona Children's Hospital, Universitat de Barcelona, Barcelona, Spain
e-mail: lucas.krauel@sjd.es; albert.pasten@sjd.es

L. Krauel (ed.), *Survival Handbook in Pediatric Surgical Oncology*,
https://doi.org/10.1007/978-3-031-65890-7_15

15.3 Clinical Presentation

15.3.1 Reasons for Consultation

Insidious abdominal pain, with or without swelling or palpable mass, is the most frequent symptom of an ovarian tumor, but other ways can lead to the finding. For example, it can be found incidentally during a routine examination, in an otherwise healthy girl [4]. Another scenario could be a finding during pediatric or gynecologic consultation due to endocrinologic changes, like precocious puberty, menstrual irregularities, or virilization. Last, acute abdominal pain could be caused by a ruptured or twisted ovarian mass, in an emergency room setting.

15.3.2 History and Examination

The age of the patient is important for a first narrowing of the differential diagnosis. It's also useful to ask about menstrual history in postpubertal adolescents and if any problem or disarrangement is occurring. Familial history could be helpful, especially when cancer predisposition conditions are present, like DICER 1 or Peutz-Jeghers syndrome, which are associated with this type of tumors [1]. History of precocious puberty and/or virilization is also important.

Physical examination could be obvious, with a palpable hypogastric mass that can rise beyond umbilicus. A fixed and hard tumor should raise the suspicion of malignancy. We could also find distension and ascites, both ominous in this setting. Genital examination may show abnormal clitoral development, pubic hair, and other signs of precocious puberty. Performing a vaginal or bimanual exploration in this age group is not generally indicated. Acne and facial hair could suggest virilization [4].

15.3.3 Further Study

15.3.3.1 Tumor Markers

Depending on the origin, every family of ovarian malignant tumors could raise one or more serum markers [5], helping to give more accuracy to the suspicion. These laboratory findings are not infallible and several times could be all negative in presence of a tumor that normally raises markers. Therefore, it is important to remark that the knowledge of these is useful, but every result must be interpreted considering the context and other findings. Table 15.2 resumes the most frequent tumor markers of clinical utility.

Table 15.2 Tumor markers of clinical use in ovarian tumors

Tumor marker	Associated tumor
β-HCG	Choriocarcinoma, embryonic carcinoma, dysgerminoma[a]
AFP	Yolk sac tumor, immature teratoma, embryonic carcinoma, Sertoli-Leydig tumor[a]
LDH	Dysgerminoma
CA-125	Epithelial tumors
Inhibin A	Granulosa cell tumor
Calcium (Ca^{++})	Sex cord stromal cell tumors

β-HCG beta-human chorionic gonadotropin, *AFP* alpha-fetoprotein, *LDH* lactate dehydrogenase
[a] Rare

15.3.4 Imaging

Abdominal ultrasound is usually the first approach to this condition, because it's accessible, fast, and safe. Its effectiveness depends on good preparation, with a full bladder for an appropriate window. Findings could vary from an uniloculated cystic-predominant adnexal mass with an echogenic nodule (Rokitansky nodule or dermoid plug), typical of a mature teratoma, to a mixed solid-liquid or solid mass, sometimes highly vascularized, bigger than the former, more typical of malignancy [6]. Table 15.3 summarizes ultrasonographic signs of malignancy.

Second-line exploration is abdominal MRI, due to its better soft tissue resolution. It's requested to perform local staging and for a better characterization of the tumor, especially when there are any tumor markers altered. In this case also should be requested a thoracic CT for rule out metastasis [7].

15.3.5 Surgical Planning

There are two possible scenarios: emergent and definitive surgeries. In the former case, the indications for surgery are adnexal torsion and peritonitis secondary for rupture or tumoral hemorrhage. When a torsion secondary to a mass is confirmed, the surgical goal is to untwist the ovary, for a definitive second-time surgery a few days later, after performing laboratory and imaging. If the tumor is ruptured or has an active bleeding, the possibility of gonadal salvage is little, and then oophorectomy is probably the safest option. If the fallopian tube has any sign of tumoral involvement, it must be removed too. The staging steps for this type of surgery (Table 15.4) should be made whether the surgical approach allows it.

Table 15.3 Ultrasonographic findings suggestive of malignancy

Size ≥8 to 10 cm
Multiple or bilateral lesions
Invasive appearance
Solid or heterogeneous: Solid nodular or papillary components (<50 percent), wall thickening, septations (>2 to 3 mm)
Increased blood flow
Calcifications
Ascites

Table 15.4 Surgical staging of ovarian tumors children's oncology group (COG)

Peritoneal fluid sampling for cytology (or washings with Ringer's lactate if there is no fluid in the cavity)
Careful inspection of peritoneal surfaces and omentum, including liver and diaphragmatic dome, with sampling of any suspicious lesion
Careful inspection of the contralateral ovary and uterus, with sampling of any suspicious lesion
Retroperitoneal lymph node inspection and palpation when it's possible, with resection of any of it enlarged

Definitive surgery must be planned carefully to minimize the risk of spread disease while seeking to preserve healthy ovarian tissue when possible. Here are two potential scenarios, too: surgery for a benign tumor and surgery for a tumor with any suspicion of malignancy.

When there is certainty about the benign condition of an ovarian tumor (negative tumor markers, imaging with any suspicion signs, asymptomatic patient), it is possible to propose a minimally invasive approach under certain conditions: a tumor less of 6–8 cm of diameter and enough experience to perform a safe manipulation of the mass, without rupture inside the peritoneal cavity. If an open approach is needed, a Küstner incision is safe and esthetically good and allows good exposure of the peritoneal cavity (Fig. 15.1).

When malignancy cannot be ruled out, our recommendation is to perform open surgery. Esthetic and postoperative benefits are less important than the potential risk of rupture and disease spreading due a minimally invasive surgery.

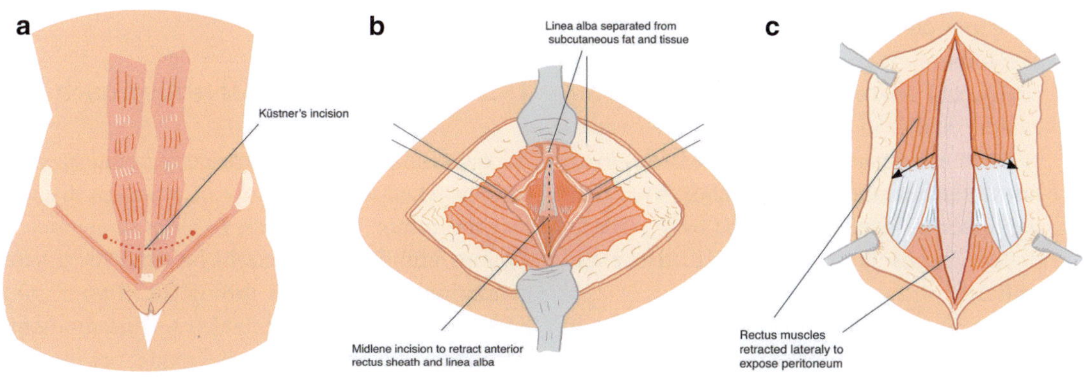

Fig. 15.1 Küstner incision for ovarian tumors. (**a**) Küstner incision at the level of the pubis depicted with a dotted line. (**b**) Anatomical landmarks after subcutaneous exposure, showing the linea alba. (**c**) Exposure of the peritoneum after lateral retraction of the rectus muscles

15.3.6 Surgical Steps for a Benign Tumor

1. The patient is placed in supine position and prepped for abdominal surgery in sterile conditions.
2. A Küstner laparotomy is made, exposing linea alba through a transverse incision, one or two fingers above the pubic symphysis. A cranial flap is constructed for further linea alba exposure. After that, the linea alba is opened longitudinally, and the peritoneum is also opened in this direction.
3. Peritoneal fluid is sampled for cytology. This step must be performed always.
4. For suprapubic approach, an elastic abdominal retractor is placed in the incision, and the tumor is carefully exposed through it, ensuring that the cystic portion can be visible.
5. The tumor surface that is visible is further protected with a plastic material, sticking it to the surface with any biological glue.
6. A suction probe is placed in the center of the tumor surface, and two silk stitches are placed there, with 1–2 cm of separation.
7. A Veress needle is connected to suction, the silk stitches are pulled up, and the needle is inserted between the stitches, while the other suction probe is placed near the needle to aspirate any drop.
8. Careful movements of the needle are made for aspirating as much liquid content as possible.
9. After aspirating, the needle is placed out and the gap is closed with a silk stitch.
10. The tumor now can be mobilized outside the cavity, and dissection is started with electrocautery marks in the line of normal ovarian parenchyma (usually is visible as white/yellow tissue near the fallopian tube). After that, the tumor is "peeled" from the ovary, like an orange, exposing normal ovarian tissue and follicles.
11. Once the tumor is removed, hemostasia in the surface is made, and the remnant ovary is closed by joining its ends, forming something like a turnover.
12. For peritoneal surface exploration, a laparoscopy could be performed through the elastic retractor, placing a surgical glove on it, and inserting a port through one of its fingers. Pneumoperitoneum is made, and careful staging is performed (Table 15.4).
13. Retractor is removed, pneumoperitoneum is drained, and wall closure by planes is performed.

15.3.7 Surgical Tips for Malignant Tumors

When malignancy is suspected, our recommendation is to do a salpingo-oophorectomy despite the surgical approach that has been selected. The contralateral ovary is inspected, and any lesions should be biopsied. If a Küstner laparotomy was selected to operate, peritoneal surface exploration could be performed with a glove, as described above (step 12 on "Surgical Steps for a Benign Tumor").

For big and solid tumors, when raise beyond the umbilicus, a better approach is a median laparotomy. In these cases, an elastic retractor and aspiration of the tumor are not necessary, but any effort should be made to prevent tumor rupture inside the cavity.

If categoric bilateral disease is found, biopsies must be taken of both ovaries without any resection, and the patient is put under neoadjuvant chemotherapy before definitive surgical resolution.

15.3.8 Minimally Invasive Approach

As mentioned above, laparoscopy could be performed when it's a certainty of a benign disease and the tumor is less than 6–8 cm of diameter. 12 mm umbilical port could be used for a safe extraction of the tumor through it. Two 5 mm ports are placed in both flanks. At this moment, peritoneal staging should be made before any other step (Table 15.4). Ovarian-sparing surgery has the same indications as open surgery and should be attempted with care. If it's risky to extract the tumor inside a bag through the umbilical port, a little Küstner or Pfannenstiel laparotomy is performed to remove the mass.

15.3.9 Complications

Maybe the worst complication is tumor rupture. If it occurs, immediate aspiration of as much liquid as possible is performed from inside the tumor and in the cavity. Unfortunately, tumor spillage upstages the patient for definition and must be declared in the surgical report for starting adjuvant chemotherapy [4].

Surgeon's Checklist

1. Ensure that the patient has been evaluated by the oncology team, and check tumor markers status.
2. See the images with the radiology team.
3. Before starting surgery for a benign tumor, ensure that you are ready to use two suction probes, Veress needle, elastic retractor or other device for protecting the wound from spillage, biologic glue, plastic transparent material, and silk suture.
4. Ensure that the incision is sufficient for a safe manipulation of the tumor. Fighting with a little incision could be very risky.
5. When a Küstner laparotomy is performed, construct a good cranial flap for a better vision of linea alba toward the umbilicus.
6. Aspirate the tumor carefully with the Veress needle. It is possible to mobilize it inside the tumor to aspirate other cystic cavities.
7. After tumor removal with peeling maneuver in benign tumors, hemostasis of the ovarian surface should be gentle to avoid damaging the follicles. A hemostatic material could be placed before closing the ovary.
8. If there is any suspicion of malignancy, or surgical findings are equivocal, perform a salpingo-oophorectomy with careful staging, take biopsies of any lesion, and finish the intervention.

References

1. van Heerden J, Tjalma WA. The multidisciplinary approach to ovarian tumours in children and adolescents. Eur J Obstetr Gynecol Reprod Biol. 2019;243:103–10.
2. Qazi SH, Jeelani SM, Dogar SA, Das JK, Saxena AK. Approaches to the management of pediatric ovarian masses in the 21st century: systematic review and meta-analysis. J Pediatr Surg. 2020;55:357–68.
3. Weil BR, Billmire DF. Management of germ cell tumors in pediatric patients. Surg Oncol Clin N Am. 2021;30:325–38.
4. Khaja A, Frazier L, Weil BR, Weldon CB, Laufer MR, Shim J. Interdisciplinary management of malignant ovarian tumors in the pediatric and adolescent age group. J Pediatr Adolesc Gynecol. 2022;35:260–4.
5. Renaud EJ, Sømme S, Islam S, Cameron DB, Gates RL, Williams RF, et al. Ovarian masses in the child and adolescent: an American pediatric surgical association outcomes and evidence-based practice committee systematic review. J Pediatr Surg. 2019;54(3):369–77.
6. Hanafy AK, Mujtaba B, Yedururi S, Jensen CT, Sanchez R, Austin MT, et al. Imaging in pediatric ovarian tumors, Abdominal Radiology, vol. 45. Springer; 2020. p. 520–36.
7. Weil B, Stark R, Billmire D, Rescorla F, Doski J. Ovarian germ cell tumors. Handbook for children with germ cell tumors; 2018. p. 7–8.

Testicular Tumors in Children

16

Lucas Krauel, Albert Pasten González,
and Tamas Prokoop

16.1 Introduction

Testicular tumors are a rare group of malignancies in childhood, constituting approximately 2% of solid pediatric malignant tumors. They exhibit two distinct peaks of incidence: one before 3 years of age and another during the postpubertal period. The characteristics and clinical behavior of these two peaks differ significantly [1]. Fortunately, testicular tumors generally have a good prognosis due to early detection and a favorable response to chemotherapy.

These tumors can be classified based on their origin. Yolk sac tumors, embryonal carcinomas, teratomas, gonadoblastomas, seminomas, choriocarcinomas, and mixed germ cell tumors are malignancies of germ cell origin [1].

In children under the age of 3, more than 80% of tumors are of germ cell origin, with benign teratomas being the most prevalent. Yolk sac tumors are the most common malignant tumors in this age group [2].

Granulosa, Leydig, and Sertoli cell tumors have a stromal origin. While stromal tumors are typically benign, they have the potential to become malignant and may produce hormones.

The second peak of incidence in testicular tumors occurs after puberty. Tumors in this age group are more likely to be malignant, resembling testicular tumors in adulthood [3].

Secondary testicular tumors (such as leukemia or lymphoma) or paratesticular tumors (such as rhabdomyosarcoma and neuroblastoma) are less frequent and can occur at any age.

16.2 Diagnosis

In most cases, the initial indication of a testicular tumor is painless unilateral swelling of the scrotum. Diagnosis is typically based on palpation, revealing a usually painless mass, sometimes accompanied by hydrocele. Hormone-producing tumors may exhibit secondary androgenization. If diagnosis is delayed, symptoms such as signs of pulmonary metastases or pelvic compression due to an intra-abdominal mass may manifest [4].

The primary tumor markers for testicular tumors are alpha-fetoprotein (AFP), beta-human chorionic gonadotropin (BHCG), and lactate dehydrogenase (LDH). Sertoli cell tumors can produce BHCG, leading to gynecomastia, while

L. Krauel (✉) · A. P. González
Pediatric Surgical Oncology, Pediatric Surgery Department, Pediatric Cancer Center Barcelona (PCCB), SJD Barcelona Children's Hospital, Universitat de Barcelona, Barcelona, Spain
e-mail: lucas.krauel@sjd.es; albert.pasten@sjd.es

T. Prokoop
Pediatric Surgical Oncology, Pediatric Surgery Department, Pediatric Center-Semmelweis University, Budapest, Hungary

L. Krauel (ed.), *Survival Handbook in Pediatric Surgical Oncology*,
https://doi.org/10.1007/978-3-031-65890-7_16

Leydig cell tumors can produce testosterone, resulting in precocious puberty. Elevated hormone levels accompany these symptoms.

Yolk sac tumors produce AFP, distinguishing them from other nonmalignant tumors in early childhood. It's essential to note that AFP levels are naturally elevated in infancy, cautioning its use as a tumor marker in this age group. Rising AFP levels in the presence of a testicular mass in early childhood are concerning.

As the initial diagnostic step, scrotal ultrasonography (US) should be conducted, aiding in the differentiation between testicular tumors and benign testicular diseases such as testicular torsion, hydrocele, torsion of the appendix testis, hematoma, or epididymitis. The US can also determine if the tumor is bilateral, cystic, or solid. In cases where US results are inconclusive, an MRI is the next recommended step [5].

An association exists between US microlithiasis and testicular tumors. However, if incidental testicular microlithiasis is observed with normal US findings and without elevated tumor markers, observation is typically sufficient [6].

CT or MRI should be performed to assess lymph node status (retroperitoneal) or the presence of distant metastases (lung, bone). Diffusion restriction in MRI can aid in distinguishing between benign and malignant intratesticular lesions.

16.3 Staging

Multiple staging and risk classification systems have been developed. Most used ones are the American Joint Committee on Cancer (AJCC) system based on tumor, nodes, metastasis, and serum markers (TNMS) (Table 16.1) and the

Table 16.1 American Joint Committee on Cancer (AJCC) system based on tumor, nodes, metastasis, and serum markers (TNMS)

T-primary tumor	N-regional LNs	M-distant metastasis	S-serum markers
P0—No evidence of primary tumor	cN0—No regional LN metastasis	M0—No distant metastasis	S0—Marker levels within normal limits
pTis—Intratubular germ cell neoplasia (carcinoma in situ)	pN0—No regional LN metastasis	M1—Distant metastasis	S1—LDH <1.5 × N and hCG (mIU/mL) <5000 and AFP (ng/mL) <1000
pT1—Tumor limited to the testis and epididymis without LVI; tumor may invade into the tunica albuginea but not the tunica vaginalis	cN1—Metastasis with an LN mass ≤2 cm or multiple LNs, none >2 cm	M1a—Nonregional nodal or pulmonary metastasis	S2 LDH 1.5–10 × N or hCG (mIU/mL) 5000–50,000 or AFP (ng/mL) 1000–10,000
pT2—Tumor limited to the testis and epididymis with LVI, or tumor extending through the tunica albuginea with involvement of the tunica vaginalis	pN1—Metastasis with an LN mass ≤2 cm and ≤5 nodes positive, none >2 cm	M1b—Distant metastasis other than to nonregional LNs and lung	S3 LDH >10 × N or hCG (mIU/mL) >50,000 or AFP (ng/mL) >10,000
pT3—Tumor invades the spermatic cord with or without LVI	cN2—Metastasis with an LN mass 2–5 cm or multiple LNs, any one >2 cm but not >5 cm		
pT4—Tumor invades the scrotum with or without LVI	pN2—Metastasis with an LN mass 2–5 cm, or >5 nodes positive, none >5 cm, or evidence of extranodal tumor Extension cN3—Metastasis with an LN mass >5 cm pN3—Metastasis with an LN mass >5 cm		

AFP alpha fetoprotein, *hCG* beta human chorionic gonadotropin, *LDH* lactate dehydrogenase, *LN* lymph node, *LVI* lymphovascular invasion, *N* normal, *c* clinical, *p* pathologic, *T* primary tumor, *N* regional lymph nodes, *M* metastasis, *S* serum tumor markers

Table 16.2 Children's Oncology Group (COG) staging system based on postsurgical extent of disease

Stage	
I	Limited to testis, completely resected by high inguinal orchiectomy; no clinical, radiographic, or histologic evidence of disease beyond the testes Patients with normal or unknown tumor markers at diagnosis must have a negative ipsilateral RPLND to confirm stage I disease if imaging demonstrates LNs >2 cm Patients who have undergone scrotal orchiectomy with high litigation of cord are stage I
II	Trans-scrotal biopsy; microscopic disease in scrotum or high in spermatic cord (<5 cm from proximal end) Failure of tumor markers to normalize or decrease with an appropriate half-life
III	Retroperitoneal LN involvement, but no visceral or extra-abdominal involvement LNs >4 cm by CT or 2–4 cm with biopsy proof
IV	Distant metastases, including the liver

Table 16.3 MaGIC risk stratification taking in consideration COG stage and age (>age 11 being higher risk)

Risk group	Stage	Age (years)
Low	I	Any
Standard 1	II–IV	<11
Standard 2 (IGCCC good risk)	II–IV	≥11
Poor (IGCCC intermediate or poor risk)	II–IV	≥11

Children's Oncology Group (COG) based on postsurgical extent of disease (Table 16.2). They differ considerably. These differences have created some challenges for collaborative trials.

Regarding risk classification, a consensus was reached to use the MaGIC risk stratification (Table 16.3) taking in consideration COG stage and age (>age 11 being higher risk) [4].

16.4 Surgical Approaches

16.4.1 Inguinal Orchiectomy

The procedure is conducted under general anesthesia with the patient in the supine position. An oblique inguinal incision, originating 2 cm superior and lateral from the pubic tubercle and extending parallel to the inguinal ligament, is meticulously performed. The subsequent steps involve the identification and careful mobilization of the spermatic cord. The vas deferens and spermatic vessels are then meticulously separated, followed by a high ligation at the level of the inguinal cord using 2–0 sutures. Closure of vessels and the vas deferens distal to the clamp is executed, culminating in division. The testis is methodically mobilized to the surgical field within the tunica vaginalis, ensuring removal with the intact tunica.

16.4.2 Testis-Sparing Surgery

This surgical approach is contemplated for prepubertal patients presenting with a testicular tumor and negative tumor markers, signifying a heightened probability of a benign tumor. It is selectively employed in cases of circumscribed tumors exhibiting well-defined borders or in situations involving bilateral tumors, where preservation of fertility is paramount [7].

16.4.3 Procedure

Under general anesthesia in the supine position, an inguinal plait incision is meticulously executed. Subsequent steps include the identification and deliberate mobilization of the spermatic cord. Separation of the vas deferens and spermatic vessels is achieved through high occlusion, utilizing an atraumatic clamp. The testis is then meticulously mobilized to the surgical field within the tunica vaginalis.

For the isolation of the testis, the following steps are meticulously executed: the tunica is opened with the cord clamped, facilitating the identification of the tumoral area for subsequent biopsy or tumor extirpation. Upon the approval of a benign tumor through frozen section analysis, the procedure advances to testis reconstruction, typically involving a 6/0 monofilament absorbable suture. The tunica is then closed.

Consideration for prosthesis replacement is viable in cases of approved malignancy.

16.4.4 Retroperitoneal Lymph Node Dissection (RPLND)

This surgical intervention is more prevalent among adult patients with testicular tumors.

In prepubertal patients (<11 years), excision of a residual mass if >2 cm should be performed when feasible, but formal RPLND is not indicated.

For postpubertal patients (≥11 years) with a residual mass >2 cm at the end of chemotherapy, they should undergo a formal RPLND [4].

The conventional bilateral retroperitoneal lymph node dissection (RPLND) approach has undergone a notable transformation, giving way to template nerve-sparing dissections for both right- and left-sided disease. This shift in technique aims at preserving sexual function and fertility, proving to be a significant advancement for the majority of patients. Remarkably, over 90 percent of men undergoing a nerve-sparing RPLND can anticipate the preservation or recovery of antegrade ejaculation. This also has been noticed to reduce operative times with equivalent surgical outcomes.

In addition to the paradigm shift in surgical approach, laparoscopic and robotic techniques have emerged as potential game-changers, offering the promise of further reducing the associated morbidity linked with RPLND, but the majority of the reports have been case series with formal comparatives studies lacking [4].

16.4.5 Metastatic Pattern in Nonseminomatous Germ Cell Tumors (NSGCTs)

The strategy for retroperitoneal lymph node dissection (RPLND) in nonseminomatous germ cell tumors (NSGCTs) is intricately guided by a well-established metastatic pattern, as evidenced by a comprehensive study involving 100 patients with pathologic stage II NSGCTs:

- Right-Sided Tumors: In 93 percent of patients, right-sided tumors demonstrated involvement of the interaortocaval nodes. This underscores the predilection for metastasis to this specific nodal region in cases of NSGCTs situated on the right side.
- Left-Sided Tumors: Contrasting with the right side, left-sided tumors exhibited metastasis to the pre- and para-aortic nodes in 88 and 86 percent of cases, respectively. This distinctive pattern highlights the regional specificity of metastatic nodal involvement based on tumor laterality.
- Stage IIA Disease: Among men with stage IIA disease, 14 percent showed involvement of ipsilateral common iliac nodes. However, suprahilar retroperitoneal lymph node involvement was a rarity in this subgroup. This nuanced understanding assists in tailoring the surgical approach based on the specific stage of the disease.
- Contralateral Node Involvement: While contralateral node involvement was infrequent in patients with early-stage disease, it exhibited a higher occurrence in those with right-sided tumors. This observation is likely attributed to the predominant right-to-left flow of lymphatic drainage, emphasizing the importance of lateralization in disease spread.
- Inguinal Node Metastases: Inguinal node metastases may occur through retrograde spread from extensive retroperitoneal nodes, scrotal invasion, or, notably, a scrotal rather than inguinal orchiectomy. Understanding

these pathways of metastasis aids in anticipating potential sites of involvement.

- Pelvic Node Involvement: The presence of pelvic node involvement may signify locally advanced disease, including epididymal involvement. Recognizing this aspect is crucial for evaluating the extent of disease progression and determining the appropriate course of intervention.

This detailed insight into the metastatic patterns informs a targeted and tailored approach to RPLND, ensuring that the surgical strategy aligns with the specific characteristics and locations of nodal involvement in NSGCTs.

16.5 Pitfalls

16.5.1 Management in Case of Incidental Diagnosis

If a testicular tumor is incidentally discovered during a testicular operation (e.g., scrotal exploration for testicular torsion), intraoperative blood samples and tumor marker labs can guide decision-making. Negative tumor marker findings may allow for testis-sparing tumor resection, while elevated markers necessitate orchiectomy. If intraoperative tumor labs are unavailable, defer tumor extirpation or orchiectomy, focusing on addressing the original operation's indication (e.g., detorsion of testes). Postoperative tumor marker labs should be conducted at the earliest opportunity.

16.5.2 Scrotal Violation

Scrotal violation occurs when any trans-scrotal operation is performed in cases of testicular tumors. Despite higher local recurrence rates, overall survival and distant recurrence rates are not significantly different from patients without scrotal violation. For Stage I tumors, hemiscrotectomy is indicated. In cases where the patient is receiving systemic chemotherapy (due to Grade III–IV tumors), further operation is generally unnecessary.

Surgeon's Checklist

1. Testicular tumors in children generally have a favorable prognosis, often aided by the early discovery facilitated by visible swelling or a palpable mass in the scrotum.
2. A comprehensive preoperative assessment includes physical examination, ultrasonography, chest CT, abdominal CT/MRI, and measurement of tumor marker levels.
3. In cases of uncertainty, MRI should be considered for a more detailed evaluation.
4. Always confirm and mark the laterality of the affected testis in consultation with the family.
5. Prior to incision, palpate the scrotum and confirm laterality with the entire operating room team.
6. Avoid scrotal violation, and consistently perform an inguinal approach for testicular tumor surgeries.
7. If uncertainty persists regarding the nature of the lesion, always consider an inguinal approach.
8. If you suspect a benign lesion, consider these steps for testis-sparing surgery: clamp the cord, take a biopsy for perioperative diagnosis, and proceed accordingly based on the findings.
9. If the patient does not require chemotherapy after scrotal violation, hemiscrotectomy should be performed.
10. Follow RPLND guidelines. Not necessary <11 years of age.

References

1. Losty PD. Pediatric surgical oncology. CRC Press; 2022.
2. Li M, Wang J, Zhang D, Hua Y, Liu F, Lu P, et al. Characteristics and outcomes of pediatric testicular yolk Sac tumor. Front Pediatr. 2022;10:1024906.
3. Taskinen S, Fagerholm R, Aronniemi J, Rintala R, Taskinen M. Testicular tumors in children and adolescents. J Pediatr Urol. 2008;4(2):134–7.
4. Aldrink JH, Glick RD, Baertschiger RM, Kulaylat AN, Lautz TB, Christison-Lagay E, Grant CN, Tracy E, Dasgupta R, Brown EG, Mattei P, Rothstein DH, Rodeberg DA, Ehrlich PF. Update on pediatric testicular germ cell tumors. J Pediatr Surg. 2022;57(4):690–9.

5. Hermann AL, L'Herminé-Coulomb A, Irtan S, Audry G, Cardoen L, Brisse HJ, et al. Imaging of pediatric testicular and Para-testicular tumors: a pictural review. Cancers (Basel). 2022;14(13).
6. Cooper ML, Kaefer M, Fan R, Rink RC, Jennings SG, Karmazyn B. Testicular microlithiasis in children and associated testicular cancer. Radiology. 2014;270(3):857–63.
7. Ghoreifi A, Djaladat H. Management of primary testicular tumor. Urol Clin North Am. 2019;46(3):333–9.

17 Extragonadal Germ Cell Tumors in Children

Vilani Kremer

17.1 Extragonadal Germ Cell Tumors

Extragonadal germ cell tumors (EGCTs) are a rare but significant tumor group that primarily affects the pediatric population and young adults. Derived from primordial cells, these tumors typically occur in the gonads (testes and ovaries). However, in about 2–5% of cases, these germ cell tumors can be found in extragonadal locations, primarily along the midline from the brain to the coccyx, when there is no evidence of a tumor in the gonads [1] .

EGCTs are a heterogeneous group of tumors with varied morphology divided into seminomatous and nonseminomatous types. In children and adolescents, nonseminomatous tumors are more common and include mature teratoma, immature teratoma, yolk sac tumor, embryonal carcinoma, germinoma, and choriocarcinoma. These tumors may also appear in mixed forms [1, 2].

In the pediatric population, EGCTs represent around 3% of tumors, with an incidence of 0.4 cases per 100,000 children. Incidence peaks are observed in children under 4 years of age, with no significant difference between males and females. Among malignant tumors, the yolk sac tumor is the most prevalent. Sacrococcygeal tumor is the most common solid tumor affecting neonates, followed by testicular tumors in patients up to 3 years of age. Extragonadal tumors can be found in various locations, including the retroperitoneum, neck, mediastinum, and, although less frequently, the vagina. Isolated cases in other locations have also been reported [3].

Unlike other age groups, EGCTs are the predominant type of tumors in the prepubertal phase, accounting for nearly two-thirds of the total cases. Among them, the sacrococcygeal tumor is the most commonly observed [1, 3].

17.2 Diagnosis

Extragonadal germline tumors should be suspected when encountering a midline tumor with heterogeneous characteristics. The symptoms can vary depending on the tumor's location. Tumor markers for extragonadal germ cell tumors play a crucial role in diagnosing and subtyping these tumors. The primary markers used are alpha-fetoprotein (AFP) and human chorionic gonadotropin beta fraction (beta-HCG). Additionally, lactic dehydrogenase, although not a specific biological marker, is essential as a prognostic factor for these tumors [1–3].

V. Kremer (✉)
Erastinho Pediatric Oncology Hospital,
Curitiba, Brazil

Clinical Hospital of the Federal University of Paraná,
Curitiba, Brazil

L. Krauel (ed.), *Survival Handbook in Pediatric Surgical Oncology*,
https://doi.org/10.1007/978-3-031-65890-7_17

17.3 Tumor Markers

Elevated levels of AFP can also be observed in liver tumors such as hepatoblastoma and hepatocellular carcinoma, as well as in rare cases of hereditary persistence of AFP with a familial inheritance pattern. AFP's half-life (T½) is approximately 5–7 days, necessitating repeated tests for suspected cases and during treatment, with intervals of at least 3 weeks. It is important to note that AFP values may slightly increase within the normal range in newborns and infants [4], which may not indicate a tumor, as observed in Table 17.1.

In addition to its elevation in extragonadal germ cell tumors, β-HCG levels may also be increased in other tumors, such as hepatoblastomas and hepatocellular carcinomas in children [2, 3]. The half-life (T½) of β-HCG is approximately 24–36 h, with a normal value typically less than 2.5 mg/mL.

Table 17.1 Alpha-fetoprotein values according to age [3]

Alpha-fetoprotein values in Newborns and Infants	
Age	Average (ng/dL)
Premature	149,700–799,800
Newborn	41,687–191,000
Newborn—2 weeks old	1500–59,000
2 weeks old—1 month old	575–5800
2 months-old	178–2000
3 months-old	88–418
4 months old	36–127
5 months old	20–46
6 months old	123–27
7 months old	11–67
8 months old	5–27
1 year old	4–17

Table 17.2 Tumor markers versus histological subtype [3]

Histological subtype	β-HCG	α-fetoprotein
Yolk sac tumor	–	+++
Choriocarcinoma	+++	–
Embryonic carcinoma	++	++
Mature teratoma	–	–
Immature teratoma	±	±
Germinoma	±	–

Lactic dehydrogenase (LDH) is not a specific tumor marker but a cellular protein expressed in various tissues, including the muscle, liver, kidney, and neural cells. Elevated LDH levels indicate heightened cellular activity, often associated with high mitotic activity in malignant neoplasms [3].

Table 17.2 provides information on the correlation between marker elevation and tumor cellularity, aiding in assessing tumor characteristics [2, 3].

The choice of imaging tests for diagnosis and the presence of symptoms will vary depending on the location of the lesion, which will now be described, focusing on the most common locations [1].

17.4 Sacrococcygeal Tumors

Sacrococcygeal tumors are rare tumors that occur in approximately 1 in 35,000 births, with a higher incidence among females (3:1 ratio). They are the most common solid tumors affecting newborns and often have teratoma-like histology at birth. These tumors typically present as a heterogeneous mass with solid and cystic components. Diagnosis can be made in utero through prenatal ultrasound or, after birth, by visualizing the gluteal region's lesion. Magnetic resonance imaging (MRI) can be performed during pregnancy to evaluate the tumor's relationship with adjacent structures and aid in differential diagnosis, such as distinguishing it from conditions like myelomeningocele. In cases of intrauterine diagnosis, it is crucial to assess tumor size and the presence of arterial shunts that may impact cardiac flow, potentially leading to severe complications like hydrops fetalis and fetal death [1–3]. In such cases, intrauterine fetal surgery may be considered for tumor resection, even if partial. After prenatal diagnosis, a planned delivery is recommended to minimize the risk involved during vaginal delivery, such as fetal dystocia, tumor rupture, and massive hemorrhage. The newborn should be evaluated for clinical stability, and surgery should be scheduled as soon as possible [3]. Tumor classification follows the Altman Criteria [5]:

- **Type I**—Predominant extrapelvic component, corresponding to 46.7% of cases.
- **Type II**—Extra- and intrapelvic component without predominance, corresponds to 34.7% of cases.
- **Type III**—Extra- and intrapelvic component, with a predominance of intrapelvic content, corresponds to 8.8% of cases.
- **Type IV**—Completely intrapelvic component, corresponding to 9.8% of cases.

The primary treatment for this type of tumor is surgical, aiming for complete resection of the lesion along with the coccyx (Fig. 17.1). Surgery can be solely realized through the sacrococcygeal region or combined with abdominal access, depending on the Altman classification. Subtypes III and IV typically require a combined approach, while in some cases, ligation of the middle sacral artery may be necessary to prevent bleeding in highly vascularized tumors; this can be achieved through either laparotomy or laparoscopy. Complete resection of the coccyx and its confirmation and radiological control afterward are essential to minimize the risk of local relapse and potential malignancy since the tumor originates from the coccyx itself. Relapsed and malignant cases are often histologically present as yolk sac tumors [2, 3].

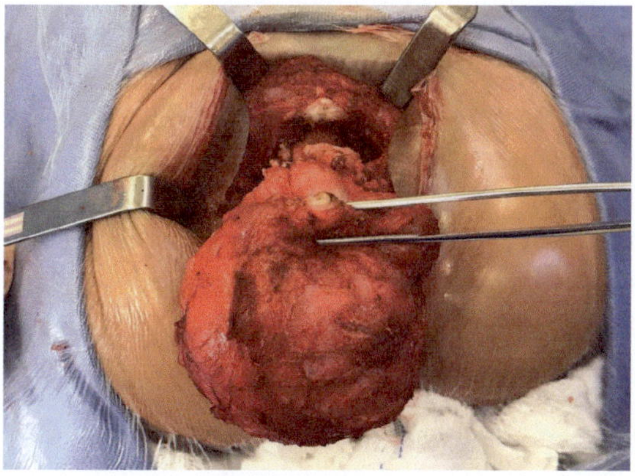

Fig. 17.1 Sacrococcygeal tumor resection with the coccyx attached to the mass

17.5 Retroperitoneum

Retroperitoneal tumors make up around 4% of EGCTs and are primarily observed in children under 5 years of age. Typical symptoms include abdominal pain, fever, weight loss, constipation, and signs of compression on nearby organs. Abdominal CT scans are used to evaluate the tumor's relationship with adjacent structures, assess resectability, and examine the appearance of the lesion. Treatment typically involves an initial biopsy or resection, followed by complementary chemotherapy.

17.6 Mediastinal Tumors

Mediastinal EGCTs are located in the anterior mediastinum and account for approximately 1–4% of malignant EGCT cases and 6–18% of all pediatric mediastinal tumors. In prepubertal patients, teratomas are the most common subtype, with a slight predominance among females. In the postpubertal phase, there is a male predominance and the presence of germinomas/seminomas or mixed EGCT subtypes. An association between EGCT in the mediastinum and Klinefelter's syndrome has been described, which should be considered and investigated. The clinical presentation can vary, with some patients being asymptomatic and the tumors being incidentally discovered during imaging examinations [1, 3].

In contrast, other patients may experience chest pain, dyspnea, cough, back pain, hemoptysis, superior vena cava syndrome, fever, and weight loss. Chest computed tomography scans can provide valuable information regarding the tumor's location and its relationship with other structures in the mediastinum and assess the resectability of the lesion. If resection is not feasible, a biopsy should be considered to determine the histology of the lesion [1]. However, if the patient shows signs of respiratory restriction due to mediastinal compression, it is necessary to consider performing a biopsy due to the anesthetic risks.

Additionally, in boys with mediastinal tumors of the EGCT type, evaluation of the testicles is crucial as the thoracic mediastinal lesion may be a metastasis from a testicular tumor, even if the primary testicular lesions are small and the mediastinal metastatic volume is large [3].

17.7 Cervical Teratoma

Cervical EGCTs are primarily teratomas and are typically diagnosed in utero or shortly after birth. Its differential diagnoses are cystic hygroma and lymphangioma; MRI can support prenatal diagnosis during pregnancy, while cervical MRI and CT scans can be performed after birth. Due to the large proportions that this type of tumor can reach, it may cause polyhydramnios, resulting in difficulties with swallowing amniotic fluid and the impossibility of breathing at birth. Therefore, when diagnosed, planned delivery by cesarean section and appropriate surgical support for the newborn should be arranged, with the possibility of emergency surgery to ensure airway clearance. One technique used in such cases involves surgical interventions and/or orotracheal intubation while the fetus continues to receive oxygen support through the umbilical cord. These procedures are called EXIT procedures (ex utero intrapartum treatment) and aim to provide necessary treatment to the newborn during childbirth. It is important to note that cervical EGCTs have a high cure rate [3].

17.8 Vaginal Tumor

Vaginal EGCT is a rare occurrence, typically observed in girls younger than 3 years of age. Common symptoms include vaginal bleeding, pelvic mass, urinary obstruction, and the presence of a tumor protruding from the vaginal introitus. Botryoid rhabdomyosarcoma of the vagina is the primary differential diagnosis, as it presents similar symptoms in the same age group. These tumors are highly malignant, and their treatment involves chemotherapy—given that mutilating radical surgery is not recommended—with excellent response to adjuvant therapy and excellent prognosis. Therefore, an initial biopsy should be performed, followed by platinum-based chemotherapy. The predominant histology corresponds to the yolk sac tumor [3].

Table 17.3 Staging of germ cell tumors by COG (children oncology group) [3]

Staging of extragonadal germ cell tumors	
Stage I	Complete resection of tumor located in a single site Associated coccyx resection, in the case of sacrococcygeal site Negative tumor margins
Stage II	Compromised microscopic margins Negative lymph nodes
Stage III	Locoregional lymph node with tumor involvement (metastases) Incomplete resection/gross residual/biopsy only with or without affected lymph nodes
Stage IV	Distant metastases, including liver metastases

The staging of extragonadal germ cell tumors is primarily based on protocols established by the Children's Oncology Group (COG), as indicated in Table 17.3.

The management of EGCTs prioritizes local control of the lesion, which, whenever feasible, is crucial for prognosis and reducing recurrences. In cases where primary tumor resection is not possible or when metastases are present, chemotherapy is initiated. The standard chemotherapy regimen includes platinum agents (cisplatin or carboplatin) and etoposide, with the addition of ifosfamide based on the extent and risk of the tumor. Most histologies exhibit good response to chemotherapy, even in advanced stages. However, for mature teratoma, which is a benign tumor, and immature teratoma, which has a low response to adjuvant therapy, chemotherapy is not recommended. In these cases, achieving local control becomes essential and is the treatment of choice [1–3, 6].

When these tumors present an increase in markers, the assessment of marker value alterations is crucial in treatment monitoring following resection or during chemotherapy. Markers are highly sensitive in detecting posttreatment relapses, allowing for early diagnosis. They also have high sensitivity for posttreatment follow-up, making an early diagnosis of relapses.

17.9 Pitfalls

A second-look approach may be necessary after treatment or during chemotherapy reassessment to determine the presence or absence of viable neoplastic cells in residual lesions. This approach is typically employed in cases where there is a partial reduction of the lesion with persistent negative markers, residual tumor with positive markers after chemotherapy, or tumor enlargement during treatment with either negative or positive markers [6].

Two specific situations warrant attention. Firstly, patients with liver metastases still exhibit a positive liver radiologic image despite treatment and negative markers. In such cases, the image of the metastasis may take time to resolve, and a surgical approach is unnecessary as long as markers remain negative and there are indications of improvement during follow-up. Secondly, when the tumor or metastasis shows growth during treatment despite negative markers, teratoma growth syndrome should be considered. This condition requires a surgical approach, and a conclusive diagnosis can be made if the entire tumor corresponds to a mature teratoma [3].

Surgeon's Checklist

1. Consider EGCT in cases of midline tumors.
2. Order imaging tests according to location (computed tomography or magnetic resonance imaging).
3. Collect markers before surgery (alpha-fetoprotein, beta HCG, LDH).
4. Evaluate the possibility of biopsy when primary resection is not possible.
5. Check if the anatomopathological exam is consistent with the preoperative markers.
6. Order imaging exams for local control after the surgical approach.
7. Check for complete resection of the coccyx after the resection of the sacrococcygeal tumor.
8. Keep oncological follow-up for teratomas as well, for they can recur and become malignant in some cases.
9. Avoid mutilating surgeries when there is a possibility of chemotherapy treatment.
10. Consider teratoma growth syndrome in case of tumor growth with negative markers.

References

1. Winter C, Zengerling F, Busch J, Heinzelbecker J, Pfister D, Ruf C, Lackner J, Albers P, Kliesch S, Schmidt S, Bokemeyer C. How to classify, diagnose, treat and follow-up extragonadal germ cell tumors? A systematic review of available evidence. World J Urol. 2022;40(12):2863–78.
2. Shaikh F, Murray MJ, Amatruda JF, Coleman N, Nicholson JC, Hale JP, Pashankar F, Stoneham SJ, Poynter JN, Olson TA, Billmire DF, Stark D, Rodriguez-Galindo C, Frazier AL. Paediatric extracranial germ-cell tumors. Lancet Oncol. 2016;17(4):e149–62.
3. Piçarro C. Capítulo 68. Fundamentos em cirurgia pediátrica. 1st ed. Santana de Parnaíba [SP]: Manole; 2021. p. 662–75.
4. Ferraro S, Panzeri A, Braga F, Panteghini M. Serum α-fetoprotein in pediatric oncology: not a children's tale. Clin Chem Lab Med. 2019;57(6):783–97.
5. Altman RP, Randolph JG, Lilly JR. Sacrococcygeal teratoma: American academy of pediatric surgical section survey-1973. J Pediatr Surg. 1974;9(3):389–98.
6. Lopes LF, et al. Protocolo EGCT-GALOP-2017 Extragonadal germ cell tumors da Infância e Adolescência. Ed Lemar, 2018.

Thyroid Tumors in Children

18

Lucas Krauel, Rosalia Carrasco Torrents,
and Maria Coronas

18.1 Introduction

Pediatric thyroid tumors present a unique set of challenges within the realm of surgical oncology. While relatively rare compared to their adult counterparts, thyroid tumors in children demand specialized attention due to distinct clinical features, diagnostic considerations, and treatment strategies due to having a higher incidence of lymph node metastasis, extrathyroidal extension and pulmonary metastasis. However, the long-term outcomes in children are better [1]. This chapter provides a comprehensive overview of thyroid tumors in the pediatric population, focusing on the surgical aspects of management within the context of pediatric surgical oncology.

L. Krauel (✉) · R. Carrasco Torrents · M. Coronas
Pediatric Surgical Oncology, Pediatric Surgery Department, Pediatric Cancer Center Barcelona (PCCB), SJD Barcelona Children's Hospital, Universitat de Barcelona, Barcelona, Spain
e-mail: lucas.krauel@sjd.es; rosalia.carrasco@sjd.es; maria.coronas@sjd.es

18.2 Epidemiology

Thyroid tumors in children are a rare occurrence, constituting a small fraction of pediatric malignancies. The incidence varies with age, gender, and geographical location. Notably, the incidence has shown an increasing trend in recent years, necessitating a heightened awareness among healthcare professionals [2]. Understanding the epidemiological landscape is crucial for early detection, risk stratification, and the development of targeted interventions.

18.3 Types of Thyroid Tumors in Children

The spectrum of thyroid tumors in pediatric patients encompasses both benign and malignant entities. The most common malignant tumors include papillary thyroid carcinoma, follicular thyroid carcinoma, medullary thyroid carcinoma, and anaplastic thyroid carcinoma [1]. Benign tumors, such as adenomas and nodular hyperplasia, are more frequent and also warrant attention (Fig. 18.1). A detailed understanding of the histopathological features is imperative for surgical planning and achieving optimal outcomes.

L. Krauel (ed.), *Survival Handbook in Pediatric Surgical Oncology*,
https://doi.org/10.1007/978-3-031-65890-7_18

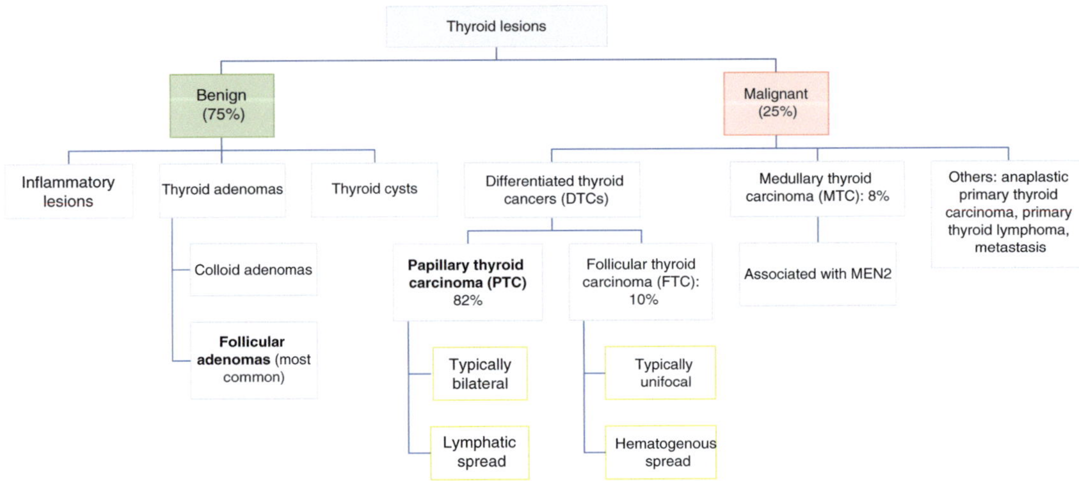

Fig. 18.1 Types of thyroid lesions in children

18.4 Clinical Presentation and Diagnostic Algorithm

The clinical presentation of thyroid tumors in children can be diverse, ranging from asymptomatic neck masses to symptoms such as dysphagia, voice changes, and cervical lymphadenopathy. Many of them are asymptomatic. Multidisciplinary management with the involvement of the pediatric endocrinologist, oncologist, and radiologist is necessary.

When suspecting a thyroid mass, basic thyroid biochemistry, tumor and thyroid markers, as well as antibodies should be analyzed. The use of ultrasound (US) is paramount as it plays a crucial role in assessing tumor characteristics, size, extension, and lymph node characteristics following Thyroid Imaging Reporting and Data System (TI-RADS) classification (Table 18.1) [3–5]. Fine-needle aspiration (FNA) biopsy is a key diagnostic tool for obtaining cytological samples, aiding in the determination of tumor type and guiding surgical decision-making (Fig. 18.2) [6]. Molecular testing, including genetic studies, may further refine the diagnostic accuracy and inform the choice of therapeutic interventions.

Table 18.1 Thyroid imaging reporting and data system (TI-RADS) scoring

	Score[a]	Risk of malignancy	Recommendations
TI-RADS 1	0–1 points	Benign	No follow-up
TI-RADS 2	2 points	Not suspicious	No FNA
TI-RADS 3	3 points	Mildly suspicious	Follow up if ≥1.5 cm FNA if ≥2.5 cm
TI-RADS 4	4–6 points	Moderately suspicious	Follow up if ≥1 cm FNA if ≥1.5
TI-RADS 5	≥7 points	Highly suspicious	Follow up if ≥0.5 cm FNA if ≥1 cm

[a]The score depends on the ultrasound nodules characteristics: composition, echogenicity, shape, margins, and echogenic foci

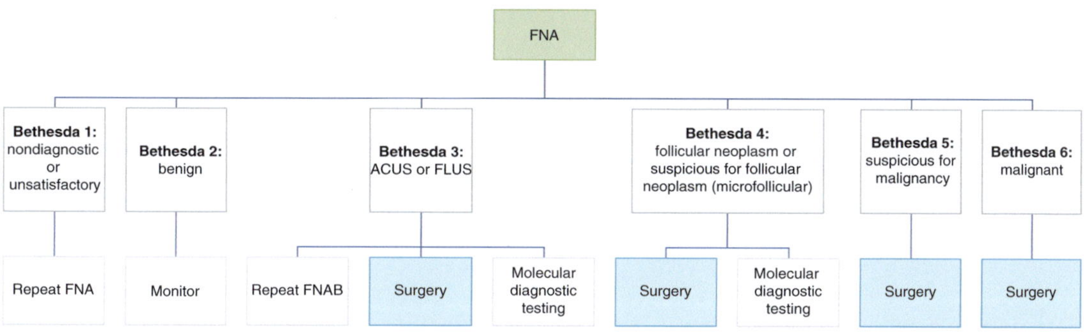

Fig. 18.2 Fine-needle aspiration biopsy and Bethesda classification

18.5 Surgical Considerations

Surgical intervention plays a central role in the management of these tumors and also in prophylactic thyroidectomy in thyroid tumor-prone syndromes (Table 18.2). In the case of patients with MEN2, the indicated time to perform prophylactic thyroidectomy depends on the codon of RET gene mutation, as shown in Table 18.3. In the rest of thyroid tumor-prone syndromes, prophylactic thyroidectomy should be performed when a thyroid nodule is detected.

The surgical approach is influenced by factors such as tumor size, location, histology, and the presence of metastasis. Total thyroidectomy is often indicated in Bethesda 5 and 6, in the presence of metastatic disease, bilateral nodularity, history of radiation exposure, and familial cases, with the goal of achieving complete resection while minimizing the risk of recurrence. On the other hand, hemithyroidectomy is preferred in Bethesda 3 and 4 [6, 7].

Table 18.2 Thyroid tumor-prone syndromes

Genetic syndrome	Genetic mutation	Predisposition to thyroid tumor
MEN2	RET	Medullary carcinoma
Familial adenomatous polyposis	APC (5q21-q22)	Papillary carcinoma
Carney	PRKAR1A (17q24.2) CNC2 (2p16)	Multinodular goiter Follicular adenoma Papillary or follicular carcinoma
DICER1	DICER1 (14q32.13)	Multinodular goiter Follicular carcinoma
Cowden syndrome	PTEN (10q23)	Multinodular goiter Follicular carcinoma
Werner syndrome	WRN/RECQL2 (8p12)	Papillary or follicular carcinoma

Table 18.3 Indication for prophylactic thyroidectomy in MEN2

Risk	Codon mutation in RET gene	Recommended age to start screening	Recommended age for prophylactic thyroidectomy
Very high	RET	–	First months of life
High	634, 883	3 years old	<5 years old
Moderate	533, 609, 611, 618, 620, 630, 666, 768, 790, 804, 891, 912	5 years old	Childhood or adolescence

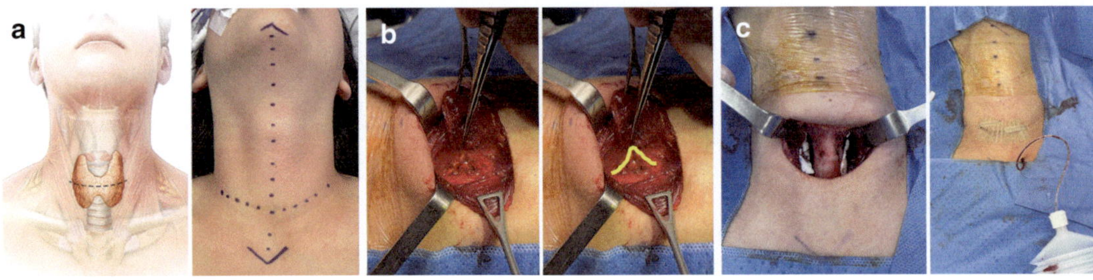

Fig. 18.3 Surgical steps. (**a**) Anatomical landmarks and incision line marked at the base of the neck, with a perpendicular incision line indicated. (**b**) Exposure of the recurrent laryngeal nerve. (**c**) Post-thyroidectomy view, showing a hemostatic patch applied on both sides of the trachea, with a drain placed after closure

Lymph node dissection should be performed in all patients with clinically or radiological enlarged central/lateral compartment lymph nodes. However, the role of prophylactic central neck lymph node dissection is a matter of debate, but it may be performed in cases of papillary carcinoma with large tumors and/or in the presence of extrathyroidal extension to address potential lymph node involvement. The prophylactic lateral neck node dissection is usually not indicated. The lymphadenectomy should be carefully planned and should be performed in a systematic way and not "berry picking." Careful consideration is given to the preservation of adjacent structures, including the recurrent laryngeal nerve (RLN) and parathyroid glands, to minimize postoperative complications [1].

In order to prevent such complications, thorough surgical planning with intraoperative nerve monitoring is mandatory. The use of new technologies for parathyroid gland preservation such as autofluorescence detection cameras or indocyanine green dye (ICG) is advised [8, 9].

Surgical steps are listed below (see Fig. 18.3):

1. General anesthesia, supine position, and neck with hyperextension.
2. A Kocher (or collar) incision is made sharply on the anterior aspect of the midneck, approximately 2–3 cm above the sternal notch, and extending between the anterior borders of both sternocleidomastoid muscles (Fig. 18.3a).
3. The platysma muscle is divided along the course of the incision with cautery. Subplatysmal flaps are then elevated to above the level of the thyroid cartilage superiorly, over the sternocleidomastoid muscles laterally, and the level of the sternal notch inferiorly.
4. The raphe between the strap muscles is opened in the midline avascular plane to expose the underlying thyroid gland.
5. In the thyroid gland dissection process, the isthmus is the starting point, and one lobe is carefully dissected from inner to outer regions across the anterior capsule.
6. Attention is given to identifying and dividing the middle thyroid vein when reaching the lobe's lateral border. The lobe is then rolled

laterally to medially to reveal its posterior capsule and the tracheoesophageal groove.
7. Superior pole vessels are dissected, ligated close to the thyroid capsule. The external branch of the superior laryngeal nerve is considered during this process.
8. Dissection continues down the lateral aspect of the thyroid lobe, mobilizing the superior pole to identify the recurrent laryngeal nerve (RLN) in the tracheoesophageal groove, protecting it through its course (Fig. 18.3b).
9. The inferior vascular pedicle is ligated, allowing the thyroid lobe to be rolled onto the anterior tracheal surface. The ligament of Berry is divided near the trachea, taking care due to being this the most common site of RLN injury.
10. The isthmus is separated from the trachea's anterior aspect, and the pyramidal lobe is resected en bloc with the thyroid.
11. For thyroid lobectomy and isthmusectomy, a harmonic scalpel is used for division, and the specimen is prepared for pathology. Total thyroidectomy involves continuing the dissection onto the contralateral lobe with gentle traction on the mobilized isthmus to expose the lobe.
12. Drains placement or the use of a hemostatic is optional. The skin is closed with subcuticular sutures for better cosmesis (Fig. 18.3c).

The surgeon's expertise in pediatric thyroid surgery is paramount to achieving optimal oncological and functional outcomes. Although there is not a consensus on the minimal number of thyroidectomies to be performed by a pediatric surgeon, 10/year seems to be the most accepted number.

18.6 Postoperative Care and Complications

Postoperative care for pediatric patients with thyroid tumors involves meticulous monitoring of thyroid function, calcium levels, and potential surgery-related complications such as bleeding or recurrent laryngeal nerve damage. Thyroid hormone replacement therapy is initiated as needed, considering the extent of thyroidectomy and the long-term impact on growth and development. Regular follow-up assessments, including imaging studies and hormonal assays, are integral to detecting recurrent disease or complications promptly [1].

Complications of pediatric thyroid surgery include hypothyroidism, hypoparathyroidism, and injury to surrounding structures. Hypothyroidism may necessitate lifelong thyroid hormone replacement, while hypoparathyroidism requires careful calcium and vitamin D supplementation. One less frequent but possible and life-threatening complication is bleeding and hematoma, which needs an emergent evacuation. A proactive and collaborative approach among healthcare providers ensures comprehensive postoperative care and timely management of complications.

18.7 Long-Term Outcomes and Quality of Life

The long-term outcomes of pediatric thyroid surgery are generally favorable, especially when appropriate surgical techniques are employed and postoperative care is diligently provided. Regular surveillance is essential to monitor for disease recurrence and address any potential late-onset complications. The impact of thyroid surgery on the quality of life of pediatric patients extends beyond the physical aspects, encompassing psychosocial well-being and familial support.

18.8 Challenges and Future Directions

Despite advancements in pediatric thyroid surgery, several challenges persist. The rarity of these tumors necessitates collaboration among medical centers to accumulate a meaningful body of evidence and refine treatment guidelines. Tailoring surgical approaches to individual patient characteristics, including age, tumor type, and genetic factors, remains an ongoing challenge.

Future directions in pediatric thyroid surgery include the exploration of targeted therapies and precision medicine. Understanding the genetic and molecular underpinnings of thyroid tumors may pave the way for novel therapeutic interventions, minimizing the need for extensive surgical procedures and reducing treatment-related morbidity. Collaborative research efforts are essential to unravel the complexities of pediatric thyroid tumors and optimize the surgical management of these cases.

18.9 Conclusion

Thyroid tumors in children present a distinctive subset of challenges within the domain of pediatric surgical oncology. A comprehensive understanding of the epidemiology, diagnostic modalities, surgical techniques, and postoperative care is essential for optimizing outcomes in this patient population. Surgeons, alongside a multidisciplinary team, play a pivotal role in the care of these patients.

Surgeon's Checklist

1. Multidisciplinary tumor board case discussion including endocrinologist, oncologist, radiologist, and pediatric surgery.
2. Make sure the endocrinologist is aware that you are performing a thyroidectomy.
3. Discuss with your anesthesiologist and neurophysiologist patient positioning and nerve monitoring electrodes positioning for reassuring not intraoperative dislodgement.
4. Mark your incision and anatomical landmarks.
5. Approaching the superior aspect of the gland is advised, and then follow down the thyroid.
6. Be aware that you will be tractioning up the gland for better exposition and dissection, but this will displace the recurrent nerve more anteriorly.
7. When in doubt about recurrent nerve location, always check with neuromonitoring before cutting. Look for another expert opinion if necessary.
8. Check parathyroid fluorescence.
9. Leave a drain if you are not sure whether to place it or not; you can even use a penrose.
10. Check postoperative calcium level (at 6 h and 24 h) and correct it if necessary.

References

1. Francis GL, Waguespack SG, Bauer AJ, Angelos P, Benvenga S, Cerutti JM, et al. Management guidelines for children with thyroid nodules and differentiated thyroid cancer. Thyroid. 2015;25(7):716–59.
2. Qian ZJ, Jin MC, Meister KD, Megwalu UC. Pediatric thyroid cancer incidence and mortality trends in the United States, 1973–2013. JAMA Otolaryngol Head Neck Surg. 2019;145(7):617–23.
3. Tessler FN, Middleton WD, Grant EG, Hoang JK, Berland LL, Teefey SA, et al. ACR thyroid imaging, reporting and data system (TI-RADS): white paper of the ACR TI-RADS committee. J Am Coll Radiol. 2017;14(5):587–95.
4. Al Nofal A, Gionfriddo MR, Javed A, Haydour Q, Brito JP, Prokop LJ, et al. Accuracy of thyroid nodule sonography for the detection of thyroid cancer in children: systematic review and meta-analysis. Clin Endocrinol. 2016;84(3):e220039.
5. Mussa A, De Andrea M, Motta M, Mormile A, Palestini N, Corrias A. Predictors of malignancy in children with thyroid nodules. J Pediatr. 2015;167(4):886–892.e1.
6. Ali SZ, Baloch ZW, Cochand-Priollet B, Schmitt FC, Vielh P, Vanderlaan PA. The 2023 Bethesda system for reporting thyroid cytopathology. Thyroid. 2023;33(9):1039–44.
7. Dedhia PH, Stoeckl EM, McDow AD, Pitt SC, Schneider DF, Sippel RS, et al. Outcomes after completion thyroidectomy versus total thyroidectomy for differentiated thyroid cancer: a single-center experience. J Surg Oncol. 2020;122(4):660–4.
8. Wang B, Zhu CR, Liu H, Yao XM, Wu J. The ability of near-infrared autofluorescence to protect parathyroid gland function during thyroid surgery: a meta-analysis. Front Endocrinol. 2021;12:714691.
9. Kim DH, Lee S, Jung J, Kim S, Kim SW, Hwang SH. Near-infrared autofluorescence-based parathyroid glands identification in the thyroidectomy or parathyroidectomy: a systematic review and meta-analysis. Langenbecks Arch Surg. 2022;407:491–9.

19 Fetal and Neonatal Tumors

Pablo Andrés Lobos and Patricio Cieri

19.1 Introduction

Neonatal tumors include a large and heterogeneous group of neoplasms that can be diagnosed from fetal screening to the first month of life. They differ from those diagnosed in older children by their anatomy, location, clinical evolution, and response to treatment. Another feature of neonatal tumors is that classical parameters of malignancy (high mitotic rate, anaplasia, and high nucleus-cytoplasm relation) can be present in benign lesions. Environmental factors are well described as a predisposing factor for cancer in adults; nevertheless they don't seem to play a role in this population. Malignant lesions can have a low invasion or metastatic progression potential, while benign tumors can be lethal due to their great size or unfavorable location [1].

As most tumors are benign, the intensity of treatment in malignant tumors can sometimes seem disproportionate. Although cancer predisposition syndromes represent less than 10% during childhood, any neoplasm during the neonatal period should raise suspicion of those entities [2]. Associated congenital anomalies, multifocal or bilateral disease, and cancer in close relatives suggest the possibility of cancer syndrome predisposition [3].

Higher diagnostic sensitivity in prenatal routine screening or in the context of genetic predisposition poses a new dilemma in the potential treatment of tumors that may regress over the first months of life. Due to the potential genetic origin of some tumors, molecular testing and genetic counseling are advisable [1].

19.2 Epidemiology

There is no actual data about the real incidence of neonatal tumors because most of the numbers are from individual institutions, and fetal death or intentional abortions are generally not listed.

Most solid tumors in this age group are benign. Incidence of malignancy is 1:12500–1:27000 live-born patients, which represents about 2% of childhood cancer. Chandrasekaran et al. published that 84% of patients with neonatal tumors were benign, being hemangiomas the most frequent. Regarding malignant lesions, neuroblastoma and congenital fibrosarcoma top the list [4]. Fifty percent of neonatal tumors are diagnosed on the first day of life. Relative incidences of neonatal tumors regarding childhood tumors are listed in Table 19.1.

P. A. Lobos (✉)
Division of Pediatric Surgery, Hospital Italiano de Buenos Aires, Instituto Universitario HIBA, Buenos Aires, Argentina
e-mail: pablo.lobos@hospitalitaliano.org.ar

P. Cieri
Hospital Italiano de Buenos Aires, Buenos Aires, Argentina
e-mail: patricio.cieri@hospitalitaliano.org.ar

L. Krauel (ed.), *Survival Handbook in Pediatric Surgical Oncology*,
https://doi.org/10.1007/978-3-031-65890-7_19

Table 19.1 Incidence of neonatal tumors in relation to childhood tumors

Type of tumor	Location	Incidence in newborns
Teratomas	Sacrococcyx, middle line, abdominal, mediastinal	35–65% of all teratomas
Hemangiomas	Skin, liver, airway, GI tract	3% of all neonatal tumors
Neuroblastoma	Adrenal glands, thorax, neck	20% of all neuroblastomas
Hepatoblastoma (HBL)	Liver	10% of all HBL
Wilms' tumor (WT)	Kidney	0.2% of all WT
Soft tissue tumors and soft tissue sarcomas	Head and neck, bladder, prostate, vagina, abdomen, thoracic wall, limbs	10–15% of all soft tissue tumors

19.3 Etiology and Genetic Predisposition

Childhood cancer may have a multifactorial origin in which genetic and environmental factors play a role. As newborns are almost never exposed to environmental factors, maternal exposure to the environment may partly explain tumor development. Presence of fetal or embryonic tissue within the tumor indicates failure in the cellular regulation during the fetal period.

According to Fernandez et al., cancer developmental factors during the first month of life are (i) genetic predisposition; (ii) prenatal exposure to maternal cancer, chemotherapy, and radiotherapy; (iii) prenatal exposure to toxins; and (iv) chromosomal anomalies [2]. Any tumor at this age should raise suspicion of a cancer-predisposing syndrome (Table 19.2) [5]. Orbach et al. show strong associations between perinatal tumors and cancer-predisposing syndromes (Table 19.2); they can occur due to high rate of de novo mutations or autosomal recessive inheritance. Confirmation of one of these tumors must lead to genetic testing in spite of no previous familiar cases [5]. If a syndrome is diagnosed, the family should be sent for genetic counseling. In cases of surgical resection, it is advisable to keep genetic material for further tests, even if the patient dies.

Table 19.2 Association between perinatal tumors and cancer-predisposing syndromes

Type of tumor	Mutated gene (DI)	Probability of genetic predisposition when being diagnosed with the tumor
Rhabdoid tumor	SMARCB1	60%
Retinoblastoma	RB1	100% of all familiar cases, 100% of bilateral cases, 10% of unilateral cases
Adrenocortical carcinoma	TP53	80%
Choroid plexus carcinoma	TP53	25–30%
Pleuropulmonary blastoma	DICER1	70%
Ovarian stromal tumors and Sertoli-Leydig tumors	DICER1	Unknown
Hepatoblastoma (HBL)	APC	5–10%
Wilms' tumor (WT)	WT1	5–10%
Medulloblastoma	SUFU	50%

DI autosomal dominant inheritance

Confirmation of a predisposing syndrome is important because of the following: (i) information can be beneficial for treatment either short or long term; (ii) a germline mutation can drive us for genetic testing in the rest of the family, especially their siblings; and (iii) genetic testing can be offered to parents seeking to prevent cancers with adult onset related to genetic syndromes [5]. Additional reason for genetic testing is to establish the probability of the same affection in a future child and help in the decision of pregnancy interruption when fetal abnormalities are found. In vitro fertilization tests can be made before egg implantation.

19.4 Diagnosis

A thorough physical exam as well as a detailed clinical history provides good information in the newborn. Ultrasound is still the gold standard in prenatal diagnosis, and indirect signs at ultrasound may include hepatosplenomegaly, polyhydramnios, hydrops, and fetal death [5].

Differentiating between a benign and malignant tumor may be difficult due to the fact that fast growth and hypervascularization are not always suggestive of malignancy at this age [5].

Fetal MRI gained popularity during the last years, especially for inconclusive (ultrasound) US studies taking into consideration that administration of gadolinium is not advisable during pregnancy. Fetal biopsy is generally not a good option, as it does not provide information that would change the therapeutic approach.

19.5 Classification

As neonatal tumors originate from fetal and neonatal anomalies, embryonal tissue, and pluripotent cells, they can have a wide distribution among the body. Expected frequency, aspect, location, and distribution may orient in the differential diagnosis (Table 19.3) [1].

19.5.1 Teratomas

They are the most frequent tumor in the neonatal period being sacrococcygeal the most common location, followed by mediastinal. Teratomas arise from pluripotent cells containing elements from 2 or 3 of the embryonic germ layers. Generally located in the midline as isolated lesions, most of them are benign at this age group and depending on their histology are classified as mature or immature.

Sacrococcygeal teratoma (SCT) is the most frequent neonatal teratoma comprising between 35 and 60% of them. The incidence is 1:35000 in live births and 30% are mature. Malignancy occurs in 10% of cases mostly as yolk sac tumor. The rest can present with immature elements. SCT presents as a visible mass between the rectum and the coccyx, and differential diagnosis with myelomeningocele can be easily made. When the mass has an intrapelvic location, diagnosis is usually delayed, presenting with urinary and or fecal retention, failure to thrive, or a palpable abdominal mass.

Ultrasound and MRI provide good information for both diagnosis and surgical planning.

Altman et al. classified SCT in four groups depending on their pelvic or abdominal location (Table 19.4).

Perinatal complications are related to the tumor size; preterm labor (polyhydramnios), tumor rupture, labor dystocia, bleeding, and high-output cardiac failure among others.

Once diagnosis is made, strict monitoring is needed to control fetal growth and early detection of potential fetal complications. Debulking fetal surgery has been proposed to prevent polyhydramnios and high-output cardiac failure. Percutaneous laser ablation of the median sacral artery has been also proposed in these complicated cases. When tumor size is greater than 5 cm, cesarean birth should be considered to avoid labor dystocia with tumor rupture and massive bleeding [1, 2].

Table 19.3 Frequency of neonatal cancer

Type of tumor	Percentage (%)
Extracranial teratomas	24–30
Neuroblastoma	23–30
Soft tissue tumors	8–12
Leukemia	6–10
CNS tumors	6–10
Renal tumors	5–7
Hepatic tumors	6
Cardiopulmonary tumors	<3

Table 19.4 Altman's classification of sacrococcygeal teratoma

Type	Characteristics
I	Predominantly external with a minimal presacral component
II	External with intrapelvic extension
III	Visible externally but predominantly pelvic and abdominal
IV	Entirely presacral

Optimal surgical outcome depends on macroscopic complete resection including coccyx avoiding tumor rupture. High recurrent rate is strongly associated with tumor rupture and incomplete resection of the coccyx. Surgical approach depends on the tumor's location. Perineal approach is used in Altman's grades I and II. When the intrapelvic component is important, a combined perineal and abdominal (open or laparoscopic) approach may be needed.

Cervical teratomas can cause hydrops due to swallowing impairment, while masses involving anterior mediastinum and neck can cause perinatal death as they collapse the upper airway. To avoid fetal asphyxia at delivery, intrapartum ex vivo treatment (EXIT) procedure has been described to assure a patent airway before umbilical cord clamping. Tumor resection while on EXIT has also been proposed.

A thorough pathologic sampling must be done searching for malignant foci (yolk sac or endodermal sinus carcinoma). If no malignancy is identified but microscopic margins are present, imaging follow-up is accepted, but the presence of any foci of malignancy is an indication for adjuvant chemotherapy. Immature teratomas do not need chemotherapy, but a close follow-up should be done as they have a higher recurrence risk. The risk of malignancy is about 10% in newborns but rises up to 75% during the first year of life [1]. Although OS is better in newborns, prenatal diagnosis carries up to 30–50% mortality. If hydrops is developed, mortality is near 100%.

19.5.2 Neuroblastoma

Neuroblastoma (NB) is the second most frequent malignant neoplasia in the neonatal period and the most frequent extracranial solid tumor overall. Derived from the neural crest cells, it can be found anywhere there is sympathetic tissue. Up to 90% of cases are located in the adrenal gland, while in older children this location drops to 30%.

Although etiology is unknown, 1–2% of the cases are family-related and have an association with the ALK gene mutation. The association to other neurocristopathies such as Hirschsprung's disease or central hypoventilation (Ondine's syndrome) is related to a PHOX2b mutation.

The advances in prenatal ultrasound findings made the visualization of adrenal masses more frequent, but differential diagnosis should be made with adrenal hemorrhage, abscess, cyst, or a renal anomaly. Prenatal findings should be completed with postnatal MRI or CT scan for a correct staging.

While asymptomatic during pregnancy, some mothers can undergo preeclampsia. Clinical course is often indolent, while diagnosis is made by palpation of an abdominal mass. Liver enlargement associated with subcutaneous bluish nodules are suggestive of metastatic disease [1, 2]. Cervical location may present with Horner's syndrome associated with iris heterochromia or paraplegia, depending on the intraspinal involvement [2].

Although almost 90% of neonatal NB have elevated urinary catecholamines (Vanillin mandelic acid (VMA) and homo vanillinic acid (HVA)), definite diagnosis is made by tissue sample (primary tumor or metastatic nodule) [2].

International Neuroblastoma Risk Group Staging System (INRGSS) staging is based on the presence of image-defined risk factors (IDRF) or distant metastases (Table 19.5). IDRF are positive when vital structures are surrounded by tumor and have been associated with more frequent surgical complications when upfront surgery is indicated [6]. In this population most NB are L1 or MS without Myc-N amplification, most of them being staged as low-risk [6].

Treatment is defined by age, biological/molecular factors, and stage. In newborns/infants observation is a valid option. In cystic lesions a nonoperative management is recom-

Table 19.5 INRGSS Staging System

Stage	Description
L1	Absence of image-defined risk factors (IDRFs)
L2	Presence of at least one IDRF
M	Presence of distant metastases
MS	Presence of distant metastases limited to the liver, skin, and/ or bone marrow (with infiltration less than 15%) in a patient younger than 18 months

mended, but sonographic follow-up is advisable. In cases when a nonoperative management is adopted and urinary catecholamines are positive, monthly ultrasounds are indicated. Tumors which don't regress or continue to grow should be resected [2].

Upfront resection is recommended in all L1 patients. L2 patients should be analyzed individually to determine whether upfront surgery or biopsy followed by neoadjuvant chemotherapy is the best option. Metastatic patients (excluding MS stage) are always treated with neoadjuvant chemotherapy.

Stage MS comprehends a singular group of patients implying a favorable outcome which allows an initial nonoperative management with clinical and imaging follow-up. In cases with tumor progression or unfavorable biological behavior, neoadjuvant chemotherapy and surgery are required. Overall survival in neonatal NB is 70–100% with 80% survival when diagnosed before the first year of life and 95% for localized tumors [2].

19.5.3 Renal Tumors

Renal tumors represent 5–7% of newborn solid tumors [1]. Around 40% are nonmalignant masses being congenital mesoblastic nephroma (CMN) around 75% of these. Wilms' tumor, rhabdoid tumor of the kidney, and clear cell sarcoma are extremely rare before 6 months of age [2, 7].

CMN is present almost exclusively in children younger than 6 months. It is generally unilateral and confined within the renal capsule. Those cases presenting early in gestation may cause significant polyhydramnios making it difficult to reach full term [8]. Although there are reported cases of local relapse and metastatic disease, nephrectomy is curative [2].

Wilms' tumor represents only 0.2% of renal tumors in newborns, and 25% of them are associated with cancer predisposition syndromes (Wilms' tumor, Aniridia, Genitourinary anomalies, mental Retardation (WAGR), Denys-Drash, Simpson-Golabi, or Beckwith-Wiedemann) [2].

Despite advances in prenatal diagnosis, only 15% of renal masses are detected during pregnancy, while 50% of undiagnosed masses are identified during postnatal physical exam.

Ultrasound reveals a characteristic anechoic rim ("ring sign") around the mass. Gold standard relies on CT or MRI and when WT is suspected, thoracic CT should be done [2].

Surgical resection of the affected kidney is the gold-standard treatment for neonatal renal tumors. In the presence of an unresectable high-grade malignant tumor or metastatic disease, neoadjuvant chemotherapy is needed. Nephron-sparing surgery should be considered in bilateral Wilms' tumor in an infant with a cancer predisposition syndrome [2].

19.5.4 Soft-Tissue Tumors

Soft-tissue tumors represent 8–10% of all neonatal tumors, being benign lesions (hemangiomas, lipomas, lipoblastoma, fibroblastic tumor), more frequently. Hemangiomas of the head and neck are by far the most frequent benign tumors at this age [1]. Multidisciplinary approach is needed for malignant tumors. Usually, biopsy for immunohistochemistry and molecular studies are important to define further treatment approach.

19.5.4.1 Lipomas

They are a type of fatty tumors formed by mature adipocytes with identical histology to normal adipocytes. With a wide distribution among the body, they can be superficial or deep (when located under superficial fascia). Lipoblastomas are rare tumors arising from embryonic white fat. They are usually located in the trunk and extremities. Complete resection is the definitive treatment, but high recurrence rate has been reported.

19.5.4.2 Fibromatosis

These are fibroblastic proliferations which are locally invasive with a high recurrence potential. They don't metastasize. Three types are described: infantile, colli, and infantile digital fibromatosis [2, 9].

Infantile fibromatosis is the most common fibrous tumor during infancy. Generally located in the head and neck as an isolated lesion, they can also present with a generalized or multicentric distribution [2]. Solitary lesions do not recur nor metastasize, being surgical resection often curative. Multicentric lesions can regress spontaneously, although bone affection is associated with higher morbidity. Generalized fibromatosis has a worst prognosis given the visceral involvement. Surgical resection is the only treatment, but recurrence is high.

Fibromatosis colli appears around 2–4 weeks of life as a localized, firm cervical mass, usually related to birth trauma. They tend to regress spontaneously.

Digital infantile fibromatosis affects exclusively the dorsal side of hands and feet. Thirty percent are congenital. Surgery is only advised for diagnostic purposes or in cases with rapid growth to avoid functional impairment, given that 60% local recurrence is seen [2].

19.5.4.3 Sarcomas

Soft-tissue sarcomas are less common in the neonatal population representing 10% of all neonatal cases. They can be associated with Li-Fraumeni syndrome or NF1. Rhabdomyosarcoma (32.8%) and congenital fibrosarcoma (24.5%) are the most common subtypes [1, 2, 9].

Fibrosarcoma is mainly located in the extremity's deep tissue (60%) followed by the trunk (25%) and head and neck (10%). As imaging characteristics may resemble those of congenital hemangiomas, biopsy is needed for diagnosis confirmation. Chromosomal translocation t (12;15) involving ETV6 and NTRK3 genes is found almost always [2]. Distant metastases are rare, and the overall survival rate is around 80–100% [3]. Upfront surgical resection is only accepted for cases where a non-mutilating complete resection can be achieved (25%) given that it is a chemosensitive tumor. In exceptional cases, limb amputation may be needed. It is mandatory to explore all available options to avoid it.

Rhabdomyosarcoma is the most common sarcoma in children although neonatal onset comprehends only 2% of them. Embryonal subtype together with head and neck and urogenital location comprises a better outcome than alveolar subtype. As they are tumors sensitive to chemo- and radiotherapy, surgical upfront resection should be left only for localized tumors smaller than 5 cm. Otherwise, incisional biopsy for histologic and molecular diagnosis is required.

Malignant rhabdoid tumors are very infrequent highly aggressive tumors. It's mainly localized in the central nervous system and kidneys. Higher rates of survival depend on complete surgical resection as they don't have a good response to systemic treatment. Overall survival is as high as 20% in the best-case scenarios [9].

19.5.4.4 Hemangiomas

These are benign vascular tumors representing the most common tumors in children, as they are present in 3% of newborns and are generally diagnosed immediately after birth or in the first days of life. Can be located anywhere among the body, and depending on the depth, they can be superficial or deep hemangiomas.

Visceral hemangiomas can be present without any skin lesion, but visceral affection must be ruled out if three or more cutaneous hemangiomas are present. Liver is the most affected organ, but the brain, GI tract, and airway may be also involved [2].

Distinction must be made between congenital and infantile hemangiomas. Main difference relies on the proliferative phase. While congenital hemangiomas grow in utero, infantile hemangiomas have their highest proliferation rate at around 12 months of age.

Congenital hemangiomas can be rapidly involuting (RICH) or present no involution at all (NICH). Another important difference with infantile hemangiomas is the fact that they are GLUT-1-negative at biopsy and do not respond to propranolol.

Diagnosis is made upon physical examination (presence of cutaneous lesions at birth), Doppler ultrasound, and contrast enhanced MRI. Biopsy should be left only for cases where radiologists can't make a correct diagnosis upon images.

Kaposiform hemangioendothelioma (KHE) is a benign but locally aggressive vascular tumor.

MRI can provide good information for a correct diagnosis, but whenever images are not clear, incisional biopsy should be taken. Frequently associated Kasabach-Merrit phenomenon consists in a severe thrombocytopenia and consumption coagulopathy. Mortality is about 20–50%, and it is determined by brain or pulmonary bleeding.

Asymptomatic hemangiomas should only be monitored by periodic Doppler ultrasound. Periorificial or visceral infantile hemangiomas can be treated with systemic or topic propranolol. Sirolimus is an m-Thor route inhibitor and became the treatment of choice for KHE. If sirolimus could not be administered, vincristine can be used.

19.5.5 Hepatic Tumors

Neonatal hepatic tumors represent about 5% of newborn tumors [1]. Most of them are benign and asymptomatic being diagnosed on prenatal ultrasound [3]. A recent paper reviewed 194 cases in which 60% were hemangiomas followed by hamartomas (20%) and hepatoblastomas (16.5%) [10]. Other infrequent malignancies reported in newborns are hepatic choriocarcinoma, malignant rhabdoid tumor, hepatic sarcomas, and MS neuroblastomas hepatic metastasis [3].

19.5.5.1 Hepatic Hemangiomas

They are the most frequent primary hepatic tumors presenting with a rapid growth a few weeks after birth with posterior spontaneous regression. Clinical and sonographic follow-up is the treatment of choice when no complications are present. In rare occasions arteriovenous shunts can lead to high-output cardiac failure, fetal hydrops, and death [1, 2]. In selected cases embolization of the hepatic artery or even hepatectomy may be needed [1].

19.5.5.2 Mesenchymal Hamartoma

Heterogeneous benign multicystic lesion containing normal hepatic tissue. Diagnosis is usually done on prenatal ultrasound screening or as an asymptomatic palpable mass during routine pediatric check-ups. Although seldom, sometimes they can be related to chromosomal abnormalities. The majority (75%) are located in the right hepatic lobe. When hamartomas become big masses, they can compress the diaphragm or vascular structures leading to fetal nonimmune hydrops and death. Surgery is the treatment of choice [1].

19.5.5.3 Hepatoblastoma

Despite the fact that it is the most common malignant liver neoplasm, only 10% of hepatoblastomas arise within the first 30 days of life [1, 2]. It is important to dose alpha-fetoprotein (AFP) serum levels and compare them with the nomogram to detect pathological levels suggestive of hepatoblastoma. It may be associated with genetic syndromes (Beckwith-Wiedemann, Li-Fraumeni, adenomatous familial polyposis, or trisomy 18). They usually are well-defined intrahepatic masses, usually lodged in the right liver. The lung is the most frequent metastatic site, and complete surgical resection is the principal prognosis factor. CT scan and MRI are needed for adequate staging. Chemotherapy is usually needed. Survival in newborns is comparable to infants and children during the same stage.

Surgeon's Checklist

1. Check prenatal imaging before deciding any surgical approach, as most lesions are benign, and some can regress spontaneously.
2. Always confirm prenatal diagnosis with postnatal imaging studies to assess correct staging and location/extension.
3. Take incisional or core needle biopsy when a tumor is suspected to be malignant and upfront resection supposes high morbidity rate.
4. Consider genetic counseling to rule out cancer syndrome predisposition and assessment for possible future pregnancies.
5. Discuss cases with the obstetrics team to define whether vaginal or cesarean birth is the best option for each patient.
6. Discuss cases in a multidisciplinary team to avoid unnecessary surgeries or procedures.

7. Emphasize physical exam to rule out/identify clinical syndromes with risk of future development of malignancy.
8. Consider intraoperative frozen section samples in small soft tissue tumors facing upfront resection with unclear margins.
9. In the resection of sacrococcygeal teratoma, especially in Altman's grades III–IV, always have in mind the possible location of the median sacral artery and how to control it.
10. Always include the coccyx in the resection of a SCT.
11. There is a growing incidence of malignant germ cell tumors in teratomas diagnosed beyond the neonatal period.

References

1. Gow K, Dellinger M. Neonatal tumors. In: Baerg J, editor. Pediatric and neonatal surgery. Intech Open; 2017. p. 65–88.
2. Fernandez K. Solid tumors in the neonatal period. NeoReviews. 2014;15:e56.
3. Merks JHM, Caron HN, Hennekam RCM. High incidence of malformation syndromes in a series of 1073 children with cancer. Am J Med Genet. 2005;134:132–43.
4. Chandraskeran A. Neonatal solid tumors. Pediatr Neonatol. 2018;59:65–70.
5. Orbach D, Sarnacki S, Brisse HJ, et al. Neonatal cancer. Lancet Oncol. 2013;14:e609–20.
6. Monclair T, Brodeur GM, Ambros PF, et al. The international neuroblastoma risk group (INRG) staging system: an INRG task force report. J Clin Oncol. 2008;27:298–303.
7. Chandler JC, Gauderer MWL. The neonate with an abdominal mass. Pediatr Clin N Am. 2004;51:979–97.
8. Tongsong T, Palangmonthip W, Chankhunaphas W, Luewan S. Prenatal course and sonographic features of congenital mesoblastic nephroma. Diagnostics. 2022;12:1951. https://doi.org/10.3390/diagnostics12081951.
9. Ferrari A, Orbach D, Sultan I, Casanova M, Bisogno G. Neonatal soft tissue sarcomas. Semin Fetal Neonatal Med. 2012;17:231–8.
10. Isaacs H Jr. Fetal and neonatal hepatic tumors. J Pediatr Surg. 2007;42:1797–803.

Rare Tumors in Children

20

Marc Wijnen and Lideke van der Steeg

20.1 Introduction

Rare tumors come in different categories:

- Typical rare pediatric tumors.
- Rare tumors irrespective of age.
- Adult-type tumors in children.

Both can be malignant, borderline, or benign. This chapter will focus on malignant tumors. The center of attention will lie on organ/location, epidemiology, biopsy requirements, neoadjuvant chemotherapy or primary surgery, possibilities for radiotherapy/immunotherapy, and additional procedures such as sentinel node [1].

20.2 Vascular Tumors

Vascular tumors exist in four categories: venous, lymphatic, and arteriovenous. These are sometimes present at birth but grow in the years/decades to follow. Treatment is with surgery, sclerosing agents, and/or serolimus. Hemangiomas, the fourth category, are not present at birth but grow rapidly up to the age of 1 year. If treatment is needed due to size or for functional or cosmetic reasons, beta-blockers are indicated. Remnants can be removed at a later age.

Hemangiomatosis is the presence of many hemangiomas also in the liver, and this is potentially lethal due to heart failure and a growing liver compromising blood flow to other organs. These patients should also be checked for hypothyroidism.

Malignant vascular tumors are hemangiosarcoma, malignant hemangioendothelioma, Kaposi's sarcoma, and hemangiopericytomas. Treatment consists of a combination of surgery, radiotherapy, and chemotherapy. Kaposi's sarcoma is associated with HIV infections [2].

20.3 Head and Neck

20.3.1 Nasopharyngeal Carcinoma

There is a peak in adolescence, and this tumor makes up 2–3% of malignant tumors in children.

The role of surgery is limited to often biopsy and debulking if needed. The mainstay of treatment is chemotherapy/radiotherapy combination. Survival is more than 90% with this combination [2, 3].

20.3.2 Salivary Gland Carcinoma

Very rare. Mostly treated with radical surgery or in combination with radiotherapy.

M. Wijnen (✉) · L. van der Steeg
Prinses Maxima Center for Pediatric Oncology, Utrecht, The Netherlands
e-mail: m.h.w.wijnen-5@prinsesmaximacentrum.nl; a.f.w.vandersteeg@prinsesmaximacentrum.nl

L. Krauel (ed.), *Survival Handbook in Pediatric Surgical Oncology*,
https://doi.org/10.1007/978-3-031-65890-7_20

20.4 Chest

20.4.1 Sternum

There is one benign condition that should always be considered when seeing a sternal tumor: this is a self-limiting sternal tumor of childhood, SELSTOC. This is a rapidly growing tumor that disappears within 6–12 months without treatment. Biopsy can often be avoided due to typical radiological findings.

20.4.2 Mediastinum

Thymomas can be benign or malignant. Both are treated with excision. In malignant cases chemotherapy and radiotherapy are often added, depending on the grade of the tumor and result of the surgery [4].

20.4.3 Lung

Most frequent but still very rare are carcinoid and pleuropulmonary blastoma.

Mostly radical excision is the treatment, but in higher-grade tumors, other treatments are added.

Pleuro pulmonal blastoma (PPB) is graded in three grades with the most solid components in grade 3. Surgery is the mainstay of treatments, though chemotherapy can be added to the treatment plan both neoadjuvant and adjuvant. The tumor is related with DICER 1 mutations [5, 6].

20.4.4 Breast

Only one third of the breast tumors arise from breast tissue, the rest from non-breast tissue (rhabdomyosarcoma) or are metastatic sites from other tumors.

Most frequent is cystosarcoma phyllodes. Malignant in 25% of cases, it is treated by local excision. A wide margin is not necessary, and oncoplastic reconstruction is not warranted if the child is not fully grown [7].

Carcinomas are extremely rare and closely related to genetic predisposition.

20.5 Abdomen

20.5.1 Peritoneal Lesions

Most often these lesions are metastatic locations of other tumors, e.g., germ cell or sarcomas.

Other malignant tumors are the following:

20.5.2 Peritoneal Mesothelioma

These present in three categories, (a) classic asbestos-related mesothelioma of adults; (b) multicystic mesothelioma, predominantly affecting the peritoneum of young women, often the prognosis is good; and (c) mesothelioma in children. Genetically the diploid type has a more malignant behavior.

Treatment is often difficult, with complete surgical resection often not possible. Hyperthermic intraperitoneal chemotherapy is a possible adjunct after an R1 resection.

20.5.3 Desmoplastic Small Blue Round-Cell Tumors

Closely related to neuroblastoma and primitive neuroectodermal tumor (PNET)/Ewing sarcoma, this is a very aggressive tumor with an aggressive behavior. The treatment is multimodal with total resection often not possible. Cis-platinum-based chemotherapy and radiation of the whole abdomen are possible. Recently hyperthermia intraperitoneal chemotherapy (HIPEC) was added to surgery with some good results reported; however, only patients without metastases to liver or lung may be eligible for this intensive treatment.

Possible targets for immunotherapy have been identified and are being tested [8].

20.5.4 Lipoblastomas and Liposarcomas

Lipoblastoma is a tumor with benign properties. Surgery is the treatment of choice with a high rate of recurrence when radical resection is achieved.

Liposarcoma is extremely rare in children especially under the age of 10 years. Resection with chemotherapy and radiation are the treatments of choice. Radiotherapy, especially preoperative radiotherapy, is a useful possibility when resection margins are small.

20.6 Gastrointestinal Tumors

20.6.1 Carcinoma of the Esophagus

This rare tumor in children seems to originate from a Barrett's esophagus. Treatment is resection, coupled with chemotherapy and radiation.

20.7 Smooth Muscle Tumors

20.7.1 Leiomyoma/Leiomyoblastoma

These are benign muscular tumors mostly occurring in the stomach, small bowel, and colon. Complete resection is the treatment of choice.

20.7.2 Leiomyosarcoma

Mostly occurring in the jejunum, half of cases are in newborns. Surgery is the treatment of choice [9].

20.7.3 Gist

Gastrointestinal stroma tumors, mostly occurring in adults, happen rarely in children. Mostly located in the stomach. Complete resection without lymphadenectomy is indicated. The treatment with imatinib is now the mainstay of medical treatment.

20.7.4 Gastric Teratoma

A benign tumor mostly occurring in boys. It has an excellent prognosis with complete resection.

20.7.5 Gastric Carcinoma

Very rare and often with delayed diagnosis, this tumor is most often lethal. Surgery seems the only treatment in localized cases.

20.8 Intestinal Polyps

20.8.1 Juvenile Polyps

These are hamartomatous in origin and benign. They may cause bleeding and rectal prolapse. Resection is the treatment of choice.

A single rectal polyp at a young age warrants a colonoscopy to exclude polyposis.

20.8.2 Generalized Juvenile Polyposis

This is characterized by the development of many (50–200) polyps in mostly the colon. 85% of cases occur in children, half of these are familial. Approximately one third will develop a malignancy before the age of 35.

Total sphincter-sparing colectomy is the treatment of choice.

20.8.3 Peutz-Jeghers Syndrome

Polyposis combined with melanin deposits in the skin and mucous membranes.

Polyps occur in the entire GI tract and start growing in the first decade of life, and 50–60% has symptoms. Resection is the only treatment option.

20.8.4 Familial Adenomatous Polyposis (FAP)

In families with FAP, colonoscopy is indicated from the age of 10. Total colectomy with rectal mucosectomy prevents the malignancy risk. The timing of this procedure is still unclear but should be around the beginning of the second decade. Duodenum should be included in the surveillance.

20.8.5 Colorectal Carcinoma

This has a very poor prognosis. A combination of late detection, high rate of metastatic disease, and often signet ring or anaplastic pathology makes this a very difficult tumor to treat.

Total resection with chemotherapy is sometimes given with good results [10].

20.8.6 Carcinoid Tumors

Occurs in the gastrointestinal tract (mostly appendix), biliary tract, ovaries, bronchi, lungs, and pancreas. Simple resection is often curative. Metastatic disease can be treated however often has late mortality, sometimes after decades.

Modern treatments include some emerging immunotherapy possibilities and Ab-based radiotherapy [11].

20.8.7 Bile Ducts

20.8.7.1 Rhabdomyosarcoma

Usually presenting with jaundice, complete primary resection is often impossible. Therefore neoadjuvant chemotherapy often makes the tumor resectable or even disappear. Radiotherapy is also an efficient therapy in these tumors.

20.8.7.2 Carcinoma

Almost always occurring in choledochal cysts, these tumors carry a poor prognosis, since resection, the only curative treatment, is often impossible, due to local progression and the presence of metastatic disease.

20.8.8 Pancreas

20.8.8.1 Pancreatoblastoma

A malignant epithelial tumor showing mainly acinar differentiation. Presenting with jaundice, abdominal mass, and pain. Diagnosis is by imaging and fine-needle aspiration (FNA) biopsy. Complete resection is curative, but there are chemotherapy regimens, and radiotherapy can be used for unresectable tumors.

20.8.9 Pseudopapillary Tumor/Papillary Cystic Tumor/Frantz Tumor

Known under different names, this tumor can occur from the age of 2 years, with a median of 22 years.

Metastases are present in rare cases, so resection of this often well-circumscribed tumor is curative in most cases. Cytology is often not conclusive, so resection on imaging is often done [12].

20.8.10 Pancreatic Ductal Adenocarcinoma

A very rare tumor, this pancreatic tumor can only be cured with total resection. So far no useful therapy is available to treat this tumor when not locally resectable or metastasized.

20.8.11 Malignant Endocrine Pancreatic Tumors

Insulinomas and gastrinomas are often metastasized when detected and are associated with MEN1 syndrome, detected by hypoglycemic episodes or excess gastrin production. Local excision is often the only means of treatment. Liver metastasis can be treated with local ablation as well.

20.9 Genito Urinary (GU) System

20.9.1 Renal Cell Carcinoma

Rare renal tumor about 6% of pediatric renal tumors. Complete resected tumors have a 60% survival rate, irresectable tumors 10%.

Resection should involve a complete resection of local lymph nodes. No other therapy is currently available; however, tyrosine kinase inhibitor (TKI) could be a new possibility [13].

20.9.2 Transitional Cell Carcinoma of the Bladder

Mostly the case in patients with augmented bladders at an early age, this tumor seems to develop about a decade after this procedure. Local resection is key and surveillance is warranted in children with bladder augmentations. Immunotherapy could be a new treatment option.

20.9.3 Cystic Partially Differentiated Nephroblastoma

This rare tumor is treated by chemotherapy and has an excellent prognosis.

20.9.4 B-Cell Non-Hodgkin Lymphoma

Although rare this tumor should always be in the differential diagnosis of a renal tumor. Biopsy is needed, when in doubt. Treatment is medical.

20.9.5 Prepubertal Testicular Tumors

Malignant tumors are rare in this age group. Mostly these benign tumors are teratomas or hamartomas. However, malignant tumors are occurring and are both yolk sac and stromal tumors. They occur in all age groups.

Treatment is surgical, in localized cases and medical with surgery in more advanced tumors. Radiotherapy has a limited role [14].

20.9.6 Melanoma

Although not a very rare tumor (comparable to Wilms' tumor in Caucasian setting), melanoma in children is still lethal in metastasized cases. Depending on the depth, resection margins should be adhered to in the (re)resection.

A sentinel node should be done to accurately stage a tumor.

With the introduction of new therapy with BRAF inhibitors, survival in metastasized patients is possible, with response rates of more than 50% and survival in 40% in adults.

The tumor seems less aggressive in children, but adjuvant chemo/BRAF inhibitors are still needed [15].

20.9.7 Target Points

Rare tumors are rare and often present late.

There are usually no standard treatments for these tumors.

Immunotherapy is sometimes the best option; always check this before surgery is done.

Check with adult colleagues with more experience with this specific tumor.

Ask for help from other surgical specialties when needed.

Surgeon's Checklist

1. Confirm with oncology, pathology, and interventional radiology to determine if a biopsy is needed and if so the amount of tissue needed and the optimal approach for the biopsy.
2. In case that no biopsy is needed but primary surgery is indicated, make sure no new treatment has become available that can make surgery easier, less complicated.
3. Obtain input from other (adult) surgeons if needed. More expertise in this tumor may be available elsewhere, e.g., with adult tumors, and orthopedic surgeons when the tumor is in the extremities.
4. Always discuss the case with a full surgical and anesthesiologic team days before the surgery.
5. Make sure you have the right equipment.
6. Pool your procedures and cluster these in one setting.
7. Make sure if a total resection is needed, or if a remnant is acceptable and can be radiated.

8. Ask for angio-CT images if needed to get a better idea of (altered) vascular anatomy.
9. Operate with the two most experienced surgeons available in a rare case.
10. Ask for (international) input on difficult cases, and reflect on the fact if the patient best of under your care, or if is there someone available who can do it better.

References

1. Carachi R. Carachi R, Grosfeld J, editors. The surgery of childhood tumors. 3rd ed. ISBN 978-3-662-48588-0
2. Atherton K, Hinen H. Vascular anomalies: other vascular tumors. Dermatol Clin. 2022;40(4):401–23. https://doi.org/10.1016/j.det.2022.06.011. Epub 2022 Sep 16.PMID: 36243428 Review
3. Qaisi M, Eid I. Pediatric head and neck malignancies. Oral Maxillofac Surg Clin North Am. 2016;28(1):11–9. https://doi.org/10.1016/j.coms.2015.07.008. PMID: 26614697 Review
4. Rossi C, Zanelli M, Sanguedolce F, Zizzo M, Palicelli A, Ricci L, Corsi M, Caprera C, Cresta C, Sollitto F, Broggi G, Caltabiano R, Cavazza A, Lococo F, Loizzi D, Ascani S. Pediatric thymoma: a review and update of the literature. Diagnostics (Basel). 2022;12(9):2205. https://doi.org/10.3390/diagnostics12092205. PMID: 36140606 Free PMC article. Review
5. Potter SL, HaDuong J, Okcu F, Wu H, Chintagumpala M, Venkatramani R. Pediatric bronchial carcinoid tumors: a case series and review of the literature. J Pediatr Hematol Oncol. 2019;41(1):67–70. https://doi.org/10.1097/MPH.0000000000001100. PMID: 29432305 Free PMC article. Review
6. Knight S, Knight T, Khan A, Murphy AJ. Current management of pleuropulmonary blastoma: a surgical perspective. Children (Basel). 2019;6(8):86. https://doi.org/10.3390/children6080086. PMID: 31349569 Free PMC article. Review
7. Knaus ME, Grabowksi JE. Pediatric breast masses: an overview of the subtypes, workup, imaging, and management. Adv Pediatr Infect Dis. 2021;68:195–209. https://doi.org/10.1016/j.yapd.2021.05.006. Epub 2021 Jun 16.PMID: 34243852 Review. No abstract available
8. Hendricks A, Boerner K, Germer CT, Wiegering A. Desmoplastic small round cell tumors: a review with focus on clinical management and therapeutic options. Cancer Treat Rev. 2021;93:102140. https://doi.org/10.1016/j.ctrv.2020.102140. Epub 2020 Dec 24.PMID: 33388539 Review
9. de Saint Aubain Somerhausen N, Fletcher CD. Leiomyosarcoma of soft tissue in children: clinicopathologic analysis of 20 cases. Am J Surg Pathol. 1999;23(7):755–63. https://doi.org/10.1097/00000478-199907000-00002. PMID: 10403297
10. Bergamaschi L, Chiaravalli S, Signoroni S, Di Bartolomeo M, Ferrari A. Management and pharmacotherapy of pediatric colorectal carcinoma: a review. Expert Opin Pharmacother. 2023;24(14):1527–35. https://doi.org/10.1080/14656566.2023.2230123. Epub 2023 Jun 29.PMID: 37358925. Review
11. Vellani SD, Nigro A, Varatharajan S, Dworkin LD, Creeden JF. Emerging immunotherapeutic and diagnostic modalities in carcinoid tumors. Molecules. 2023;28(5):2047. https://doi.org/10.3390/molecules28052047. PMID: 36903295 Free PMC article. Review
12. Campanile M, Nicolas A, LeBel S, Delarue A, Guys JM, de Lagausie P. Frantz's tumor: is mutilating surgery always justified in young patients? Surg Oncol. 2011;20(2):121–5. https://doi.org/10.1016/j.suronc.2009.12.003. Epub 2010 Jan 27.PMID: 20106656. Review
13. Craig KM, Poppas DP, Akhavan A. Pediatric renal cell carcinoma. Curr Opin Urol. 2019;29(5):500–4. https://doi.org/10.1097/MOU.0000000000000656. PMID: 31261184 Review
14. Aldrink JH, Glick RD, Baertschiger RM, Kulaylat AN, Lautz TB, Christison-Lagay E, Grant CN, Tracy E, Dasgupta R, Brown EG, Mattei P, Rothstein DH, Rodeberg DA, Ehrlich PF. Update on pediatric testicular germ cell tumors. J Pediatr Surg. 2022;57(4):690–9. https://doi.org/10.1016/j.jpedsurg.2021.04.001. Epub 2021 Apr 15.PMID: 33975708 Review
15. Pampena R, Piccolo V, Muscianese M, Kyrgidis A, Lai M, Russo T, Briatico G, Di Brizzi EV, Cascone G, Pellerone S, Longo C, Moscarella E, Argenziano G. Melanoma in children: a systematic review and individual patient meta-analysis. J Eur Acad Dermatol Venereol. 2023;37(9):1758–76. https://doi.org/10.1111/jdv.19220. Epub 2023 Jun 2.PMID: 37210654 Review

The Role of the Pediatric Surgeon in Bone Tumors: Thoracic Ewing Sarcoma and Osteosarcomas

21

Alessandro Crocoli, Giorgio Persano, Cristina Martucci, Silvia Madafferi, and Alessandro Inserra

21.1 Introduction

Osteosarcoma is the most prevalent primary malignant bone tumor in adolescents and young adults under 20 years old, with approximately 10,000 cases per year. The age distribution is bimodal, with a peak during adolescence and a second peak in older individuals [1]. Multimodality therapy has improved prognosis for adolescents with bone and soft tissue sarcomas, and routine multi-agent chemotherapy has reduced the risk of metastatic disease. Local tumor control is crucial for pediatric patients with certain sarcomas, as it eliminates the source of clonogenic cells and preserves the primary tumor site's function. Factors contributing to increased local control effectiveness include three-dimensional imaging, new radiation therapy modalities, surgical reconstructive techniques, and new chemotherapeutic agents. Ewing tumors are rare and difficult to categorize, with bone tumor incidence rates in children being 2.9 per million and soft tissue localization rates at 0.4 per million.

A. Crocoli (✉) · G. Persano · C. Martucci · S. Madafferi · A. Inserra
Surgical Oncology Unit, Bambino Gesù Children Hospital IRCCS, Rome, Italy
e-mail: alessandro.crocoli@opbg.net; giorgio.persano@opbg.net; cristina.martucci@opbg.net; silvia.madafferi@opbg.net; alessandro.inserra@opbg.net

21.2 General Principles

Surgical indications for the treatment of sarcomas include initial biopsies, resection of the primary tumor, reconstruction following resection, and, in some cases, resection of metastatic lesions. Several of these topics will be discussed in greater depth for each disease, but some general principles that apply to all of them are enumerated below.

21.2.1 Biopsy

Biopsy principles include longitudinal incisions, surgical excision of the biopsy tract, avoidance of neurovascular structures, and direct tumor access through muscles. Open incisional biopsy is recommended for minors to obtain sufficient tissue for biological studies. A minimum of 1 cm^3 of tissue is required for cytogenetic, molecular, and immunohistochemistry analyses. Bone tumors can be diagnosed by biopsy, avoiding breaking weakened bones and increasing the risk of fractures. The treatment approach is optimized through collaboration between pediatric oncologists, radiation oncologists, and surgeons for accurate staging before local therapy. Patients undergoing unanticipated surgical excision of a "mass" are at increased risk for local recurrence and loss of function [2].

L. Krauel (ed.), *Survival Handbook in Pediatric Surgical Oncology*,
https://doi.org/10.1007/978-3-031-65890-7_21

21.2.2 Surgical Guidelines

Enneking et al. have identified surgical margins as radical, wide, marginal, and intralesional options [3]. A radical margin involves the complete removal of a muscle compartment containing a tumor, which is rare for sarcoma. A wide margin is obtained when the tumor is removed in its entirety, but this may leave microscopic residual disease. An intralesional margin, or debulking, exposes the tumor during surgery, contaminating the operative field and leaving a gross macroscopic tumor behind.

A large surgical margin is crucial for local control of sarcomas during surgery. Factors such as the presence of other essential structures and the type of tissue close to the tumor's edge determine the margin's sufficiency. Thick fascial connective tissue is considered an acceptable margin even if it is extremely close to the tumor. Margins are typically closest near neurovascular structures, with major nerves like the femoral being sacrificed for functional results.

Surgery may struggle to obtain wide margins in certain anatomic regions due to the proximity of important structures to the tumor. Neoadjuvant chemotherapy may be administered to chemotherapy-sensitive cancers to reduce the size of the tumor or reactive zone if a broad surgical margin is not achieved. For some patients, radiation may be necessary before or after surgery to achieve desired local control.

21.2.3 Incomplete Excisions

Incomplete sarcoma removal, often due to not being suspected at the time of surgery, is recommended. Current incomplete excision rates range from 18% to 53%, with 30% reported in most studies. Re-excision of the contaminated sarcoma bed and adjuvant radiation therapy may be necessary depending on the lesion's location. Without re-excision, recurrence rates for sarcomas with positive margins can range from 70% to 90%. Microscopic disease is observed in 14% to 74% of re-excised tumor specimens. Re-excision is typically associated with increased morbidity during surgery [4].

21.2.4 Osteosarcoma

Osteosarcoma requires effective systemic chemotherapy and complete surgical resection, preferably with wide margins, of all clinically detectable disease, including metastatic sites. Surgery is the mainstay of local control, as osteosarcoma is unresponsive to radiotherapy. To prevent local recurrence, all gross and microscopic tumors must be removed along with a circle of normal tissue. Primary surgical procedures include amputation and limb salvage, with the fundamental principle of en bloc excision through normal tissue planes. Most patients with osteosarcoma undergo induction chemotherapy before definitive surgical resection. Factors such as tumor location, size, relationship to adjacent neurovascular structures, patient's age and skeletal maturity, reconstruction possibility, and necrosis estimate are considered [5]. There is no survival disadvantage for carefully selected patients treated by experienced surgeons with limb-saving procedures. Patients with narrow margins and poor histologic response to presurgical chemotherapy have a higher risk of local recurrence. Amputation is necessary if complete excision cannot be achieved or if resection margins are positive. Patients with osteosarcoma of the axial skeleton face challenges in obtaining wide resection margins [4, 6].

21.3 Ewing Sarcoma

Prior to the development of chemotherapy in the 1970s, only 10% of individuals diagnosed with Ewing's sarcoma were expected to survive. Radiation therapy became the primary treatment for the immediate area, but surgery has been reintroduced due to advancements in surgical methods, neoadjuvant chemotherapy, and increased oncologic training [7].

Surgical removal of tumors has two primary advantages: lower rates of local failure and increased survival chances and the possibility of researching how neoadjuvant chemotherapy inhibits tumor growth. The pathologic response of these tumors to chemotherapy can provide insight into the patient's prognosis, making surgery the most common method for achieving local control [8, 9].

Certifications favor surgery as a method for achieving local control include small initial tumor volume, location in an expendable bone, tumors in the diaphysis, and tumors that have a good response to chemotherapy. Diaphyseal resections offer the greatest potential for functional improvement, and limb-sparing surgical operations are no longer considered medically inappropriate for patients with pathologic fractures.

However, dealing with very young children presents additional problems, as local management of long bones results in reduced future limb growth and a difficult-to-maintain limb length discrepancy. In some cases, achieving a wide surgical margin may require excising a portion of the joint surface, narrowing the range of possible reconstructions for children under 10 years old.

21.4 Chest Wall

The resection of chest wall sarcomas typically follows the rule of thumb that 4 cm margins are required for high-grade lesions, while low-grade lesions only require 2 cm margins. However, there is limited evidence to support this general rule of thumb. A single-center retrospective series conducted at the Mayo Clinic found that a margin of more than 4 cm was related with a 5-year survival rate of 56%, whereas a margin of just 2 cm was associated with a survival rate of 29%. This study did not consider tumor size, grade, or histology, and it also did not approach statistical significance [10, 11].

A more recent study by Shewale et al. [12] followed 121 patients diagnosed with primary chest wall sarcoma over the course of 15 years. They found that R0 resection was an independent predictor of survival after chest wall resection (HR 5.6; 95% CI 2.95–11.93; P.001) [12]. In a 2015 study, researchers looked at the outcomes of 65 cases of chest wall sarcoma (excluding Ewing sarcoma and chondrosarcoma histologies) and found that patients with stage IIb and stage III disease had a lower risk of local recurrence and distant metastases when they received radiation therapy and chemotherapy, respectively, at 5- and 10-year endpoints [13].

There is a dearth of data on long-term functional outcomes in the chest population, in contrast to the orthopedic group, which is extremely well defined. This presents an additional barrier, making it impossible to conduct a risk-benefit analysis of radical resections. Therefore, there is no data that strongly indicates a modification in the universally established practice of resecting chest wall tumors at a depth of 2 cm for low-grade tumors and 4 cm for high-grade tumors.

For bone sarcoma excision, a negative surgical margin has been cited as a key factor in determining the likelihood of local recurrence and overall survival. Literature suggests that tumor necrosis following neoadjuvant chemotherapy and pleural involvement may be predictive of overall survival outcome. However, due to the rarity of this histology, previous studies lacked the statistical power to definitively answer the question of which factors are clearly associated with overall survival [10].

Osteosarcoma is typically a histology for which surgery and chemotherapy are the primary treatments. When surgery and chemotherapy are combined to treat skeletal osteosarcoma, survival is typically improved. With osteosarcoma, the function of radiation therapy is generally reserved for palliative situations, as it is more controversial. Radiation-induced sarcomas (RIS) typically develop following radiation to the chest wall for breast cancer, lung cancer, or non-Hodgkin lymphoma, with a minimum latency period of 3 years and a median latency period of 10–15 years. Wide excision is the treatment of choice for RIS of the chest wall, with a relatively poor prognosis for local recurrence and overall survival.

21.5 Surgical Reconstruction

The literature contains extensive single-center case series from prestigious institutions, including the Mayo Clinic, Emory University, Memorial Sloan Kettering, and MD Anderson Cancer Center, which are considered authoritative on this subject. Each center has developed a unique and nuanced approach with some overlapping similarities, but there is no general consensus or clear superiority regarding many of the technical aspects, such as the type of mesh to implant or the use of rigid versus flexible prostheses for chest wall stabilization.

There is widespread consensus that the fundamental guiding principles for chest wall reconstruction should be to stabilize the thorax in order to accomplish:

1. Optimal respiratory function.
2. Protection of underlying organs.
3. An acceptable cosmetic outcome. A multidisciplinary approach is required for these frequently complex patients.

The plan for thoracic wall resection will ultimately be influenced by surgeon preference and available resources.

Reconstruction required?

Certain thoracic wall defects do not always necessitate reconstruction. The two main, interrelated factors are defect size and location. Numerous researchers concur that reconstruction is not required for defects smaller than 5 cm in any location, or up to 10 cm if protected by the scapula, and there is no danger of scapular entrapment. The so-called critical areas of the chest that require skeletal reconstruction are the anterior or lateral chest wall and the absence of three or more ribs covered by the scapula. Without reconstruction in a critical area, 100% of patients experienced respiratory complications, compared to patients who underwent reconstruction.

Should flexible or unyielding material be used?

The ideal characteristics of a prosthesis include:

- Sufficient stability to eliminate paradoxical chest movement.
- Malleability to permit shaping.
- The capacity for host tissue ingrowth/incorporation.
- Resistance to infection.
- Radiolucence.
- Cost tolerance.
- Durability with long-term mechanical integrity.

In addition, the choice of prosthesis is crucial to the concept of "biomimesis," in which the natural biological form and function of the chest wall are replicated.

The only definitive conclusions that can be drawn from the literature are that there is presently no perfect prosthetic material and that any type of prosthetic material (rigid or flexible) can be used successfully in the hands of a skilled practitioner.

Flexible materials are the simplest to implant, but rigidity, which is optimal for preserving respiratory mechanics, is sacrificed. The ability of porous materials to support tissue ingrowth appears to confer greater resistance to infection. In the experience of the authors, the absence of tissue incorporation of polytetrafluoroethylene (PTFE) increases the frequency of infection reintervention. Methacrylate is the most commonly used material for rigid chest wall reconstruction [10]. The fabrication of a methacrylate composite with a porous mesh enables customized solutions. Similar to PTFE, methacrylate does not integrate into the surrounding tissue, increasing the danger of wound seroma and infection. 10% to 20% of patients with methacrylate prostheses report wound complications; 5% ultimately necessitate prosthesis removal. Additionally, the rigidity of methacrylate can be problematic in environments with a dynamic chest wall. This can result in stress fractures and breathing discomfort. Titanium mesh plate alternatives for rigid chest wall reconstruction are gaining popularity. Notably, these uses remain "off-label" and should be approached with caution. Plating systems for the ribs, for example, are typically limited to traversing relatively small unsupported bone openings. Unknown is the long-term stability and durability of plates placed over significant bone gaps.

Surgeon's Checklist
Osteosarcoma

1. The purpose of surgery is to remove the tumor with adequate surgical margins while preserving the optimal function of the operated part.
2. When the entire tumor is excised with extensive or radical margins, surgery is deemed effective. The margins of surgical excision must be determined through close collaboration between the surgeon and pathologist. In the case of macroscopic residues, the ultimate evaluation of the surgical margins may necessitate additional interventions up to and including amputation.
3. According to the Enneking classification [3], surgical margins are radical, wide, marginal, intralesional, and contaminated.
4. The surgical treatment of pulmonary metastases is recommended if preoperative chemotherapy results in a response or disease stability.
5. In the case of disease progression or extrapulmonary disease that is not amenable to surgical therapy, surgical treatment of pulmonary metastases is not advised.
6. The standard treatment for isolated pulmonary metastases is surgery. Free range, number of nodules, and resectability are the primary prognostic factors for these patients. In the case of unilateral metastases, there is no evidence that a surgical approach that permits palpation of the contralateral lung provides a survival benefit. Wherever technically practicable, repeated metastasectomy is always advised in cases of pulmonary metastases.
7. In all situations where a complete surgical excision of the metastatic disease is possible, metastatic surgery is recommended for symptomatic metastases. The surgical strategy must always prioritize conservative treatments and the patient's quality of life.

Ewing Sarcoma

1. Surgery is the recommended local treatment for Ewing's sarcoma whenever feasible. The goal of surgery is to remove the tumor with wide margins while preserving the best functional recovery.
2. According to the Enneking classification, surgical margins are radical, wide, marginal, intralesional, and contaminated. The margins of surgical excision must be determined through close collaboration between the surgeon and pathologist. There is a strong correlation between surgical margin quality and the risk of local recurrence.
3. For the purposes of any postoperative radiotherapy treatment, titanium clips should be used to mark areas with "risky" margins identified during the surgical procedure.

References

1. Smeland S, Bielack SS, Whelan J, Bernstein M, Hogendoorn P, Krailo MD, et al. Survival and prognosis with osteosarcoma: outcomes in more than 2000 patients in the EURAMOS-1 (European and American osteosarcoma study) cohort. Eur J Cancer. 2019;109:36–50. https://doi.org/10.1016/j.ejca.2018.11.027.
2. Ferguson JL, Turner SP. Bone cancer: diagnosis and treatment principles. Am Fam Physician. 2018;98(4):205–13.
3. Enneking WF, Spanier SS, Goodman MA. A system for the surgical staging of musculoskeletal sarcoma. Clin Orthop Relat Res. 1980;2003(415):4–18. https://doi.org/10.1097/01.blo.0000093891.12372.0f.
4. Kawaguchi N, Ahmed AR, Matsumoto S, Manabe J, Matsushita Y. The concept of curative margin in surgery for bone and soft tissue sarcoma. Clin Orthop Relat Res. 2004;419:165–72. https://doi.org/10.1097/00003086-200402000-00027.
5. Isakoff MS, Bielack S, Meltzer P, Gorlick R. Osteosarcoma: current treatment and a collaborative pathway to success. J Clin Oncol. 2015;33(27):3029–35. https://doi.org/10.1200/jco.2014.59.4895.
6. Grimer R. Surgical options for children with osteosarcoma. Lancet Oncol. 2005;6(2):85–92. https://doi.org/10.1016/S1470-2045(05)01734-1.
7. Biswas B, Rastogi S, Khan SA, Mohanti BK, Sharma DN, Sharma MC, et al. Outcomes and prognostic factors for Ewing-family tumors of the extremities. J Bone Joint Surg Am. 2014;96(10):841–9. https://doi.org/10.2106/JBJS.M.00411.
8. Reed DR, Hayashi M, Wagner L, Binitie O, Steppan DA, Brohl AS, et al. Treatment pathway of bone sarcoma in children, adolescents, and young adults. Cancer. 2017;123(12):2206–18. https://doi.org/10.1002/cncr.30589.
9. Williams AK, Crawford B, Federman NC, Bernthal N, Arkader A. What's new in pediatric orthopaedic

tumor surgery. J Pediatr Orthop. 2021;41(2):e174–80. https://doi.org/10.1097/BPO.0000000000001689.
10. Sandler G, Hayes-Jordan A. Chest wall reconstruction after tumor resection. Semin Pediatr Surg. 2018;27(3):200–6. https://doi.org/10.1053/j.sempedsurg.2018.05.008.
11. Scarnecchia E, Liparulo V, Capozzi R, Ceccarelli S, Puma F, Vannucci J. Chest wall resection and reconstruction for tumors: analysis of oncological and functional outcome. J Thorac Dis. 2018;10(Suppl 16):S1855–63. https://doi.org/10.21037/jtd.2018.05.191.
12. Shewale JB, Mitchell KG, Nelson DB, Conley AP, Rice DC, Antonoff MB, et al. Predictors of survival after resection of primary sarcomas of the chest wall-A large, single-institution series. J Surg Oncol. 2018;118(3):518–24. https://doi.org/10.1002/jso.25162.
13. Burt A, Berriochoa J, Korpak A, Rodler E, Jones RL, Weisstein J, et al. Treatment of chest wall sarcomas: a single-institution experience over 20 years. Am J Clin Oncol. 2015;38(1):80–6. https://doi.org/10.1097/COC.0b013e31828aac22.

General Surgical Emergencies in the Pediatric Oncologic Patient

22

Elena Weigl, Kristina Lisec, Beate Häberle, and Oliver J. Muensterer

22.1 Introduction

Since pediatric oncologic patients tend to undergo prolonged and intensive therapies, they are not only prone to therapy-associated risks and comorbidities, but they remain liable for all types of general pediatric emergencies as well. The underlying disease itself, as well as the oncologic therapy, may influence the presenting symptoms, which in turn can delay diagnosis. Patients with neutropenia and malnutrition, as well as those who underwent radiotherapy, steroid therapy, or chemotherapy, are at a high risk for infections and delayed wound healing. All of these factors are associated with higher morbidity and mortality following surgery [1, 2]. It is therefore crucial to keep a high index of suspicion regarding symptom interpretation. Individual treatment plans should be discussed in an interdisciplinary setting, as standard procedures can turn into life-threatening interventions in neutropenic oncologic patients.

E. Weigl · K. Lisec · B. Häberle · O. J. Muensterer (✉)
Department of Pediatric Surgery, Dr. von Hauner Children's Hospital, LMU Medical Center, Munich, Germany
e-mail: Elena.Weigl@med.uni-muenchen.de; Kristina.Lisec@med.uni-muenchen.de; Beate.Haeberle@med.uni-muenchen.de; oliver.muensterer@med.uni-muenchen.de

22.2 General Considerations

Trauma and injury are the most common causes for emergency department consultations in children. In bone marrow-suppressed patients, even minor trauma can lead to prolonged bleeding and extensive blood loss. However, other surgical emergencies require special considerations as well. When treating general pediatric surgical emergencies, risks and benefits need to be weighed against each other with particular attention. Mortality from abdominal emergency surgery has been shown to be 12-fold higher compared to mortality for elective operations in neutropenic patients [1]. If an operative intervention is unavoidable and cannot be postponed, potential risk factors should be identified and addressed preoperatively. This includes preferentially performing surgery in a center with ample experience regarding the condition and interdisciplinary care by both the pediatric surgeon and the pediatric oncologist. In some cases, a minimal-invasive approach may decrease the risk of wound complications. The timing of the operative procedure is also important, as bloodstream infections increase during the 7 days following chemotherapy [2]. Thrombocytopenia and other coagulopathies should be corrected before an operative procedure, including the pausation of ongoing antithrombotic prophylaxis. Perioperative antibiotic therapy should be liberally considered.

L. Krauel (ed.), *Survival Handbook in Pediatric Surgical Oncology*,
https://doi.org/10.1007/978-3-031-65890-7_22

There is no reported higher risk for deep venous thrombosis in children with cancer, albeit cancer being a risk factor in itself. Therefore, routine postoperative antithrombotic prophylaxis is not recommended [2]. Although usually avoided in children, non-resorbable sutures should be considered in patients with delayed wound healing since they may remain in situ longer than usual and may predispose to infection. Tertiary wound closure, or vacuum-assisted wound closure, may be necessary in infectious settings [1]. Figure 22.1 provides a flowchart for individual decision-making, as well as an exemplary preoperative checklist.

22.3 Abdominal Pain

Abdominal pain and vomiting in immunocompromised children may result from a variety of reasons [1]. A broad diagnostic differential must be considered, ranging from chemotherapy-induced side effects to general pediatric illnesses (Fig. 22.2). The workup of such patients can be

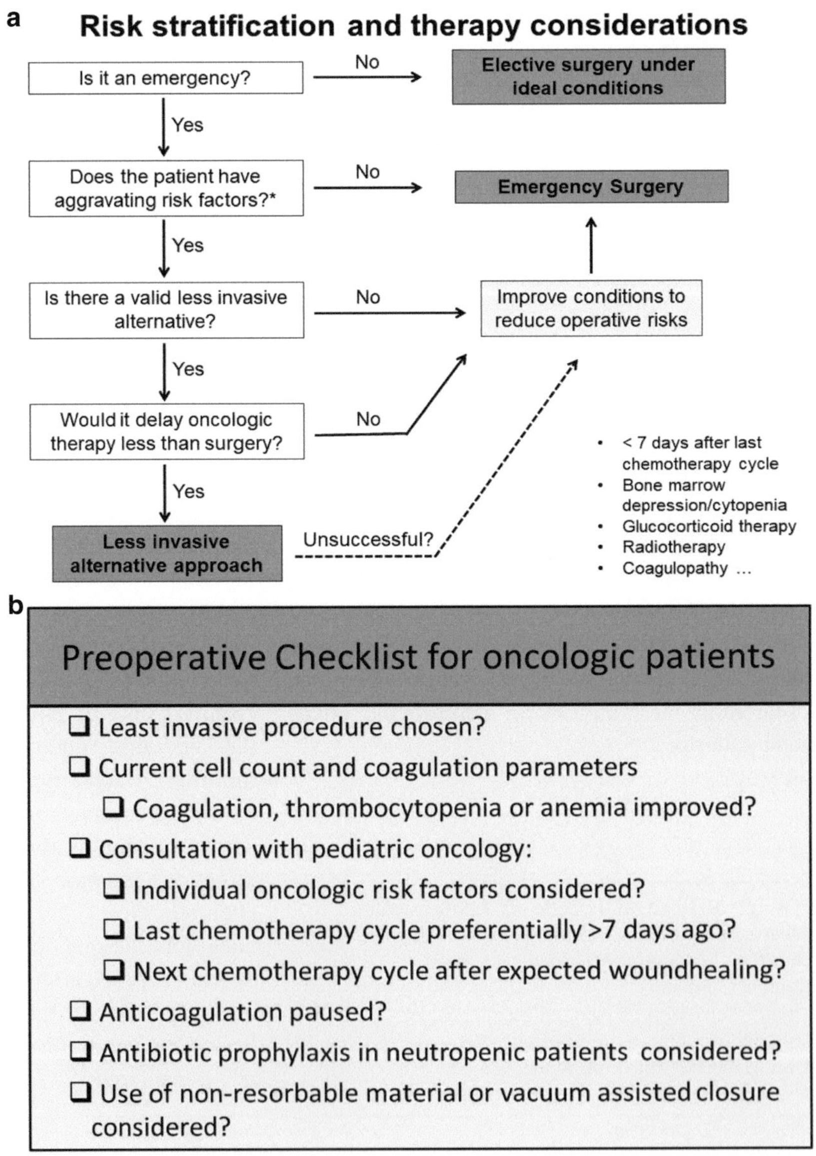

Fig. 22.1 General considerations for surgical emergencies in the pediatric oncologic patient. Algorithm for surgical intervention (**a**) and on-call checklist for the consulted pediatric surgeon (**b**)

Abdominal pain in pediatric cancer patients

• Appendicits	• Pancreatitis
• Neutropenic colitis/ typhlitis	• Infectious gastroenteritis
• Ischemic colitis	• Intussusception
• Chemotherapy associated mucositis	• Cholangitis
• Veno-occlusive disease	• Cholecystitis
• Medication induced ileus	• Graft versus Host disease

Fig. 22.2 Differential diagnosis of abdominal pain in pediatric cancer patients

challenging, as laboratory findings and clinical symptoms may be modulated by associated therapies and underlying conditions. A definitive diagnosis is only established intraoperatively in about half of oncologic patients, and up to a third of cases remain cryptic [1]. Specific imaging is generally helpful to make the diagnosis. Since ultrasound studies are very operator-dependent, a computed tomography or magnetic resonance imaging examination should be performed in unclear cases. Endoscopy has a higher risk for perforation in oncologic patients and is therefore discouraged [3]. Blood cultures and microbiological analyses should be obtained to guide antibiotic therapy.

22.4 Acute Appendicitis

Acute appendicitis is the most common indication for abdominal surgery in children, and oncologic patients may be affected as well. Pediatric cancer patients presenting with abdominal pain in the right lower quadrant should always be evaluated for acute appendicitis, as early diagnosis is essential due to the possibility of rapid progression. Appendiceal perforation is a major risk factor for prolonged hospitalization and delay in further oncologic treatment, as drainage or surgery may be indicated. The most common cause for death of neutropenic patients after abdominal emergency surgery is sepsis. Therefore, an early nonoperative approach with antibiotics, bowel rest, bone marrow growth factor stimulation, as well as drainage of a fluid collection is recommended in stable neutropenic patients. The risks and benefits of an operative approach should be weighed carefully, as mortality in emergency abdominal surgery has been reported in up to 16.4% of neutropenic patients [1]. However, a retrospective study found that upfront appendectomy in children with neutropenic appendicitis compared to nonoperative treatment may be associated with fewer complications, shorter hospital stay, and lower needs of postponing chemotherapy [4].

22.5 Neutropenic Enterocolitis

Neutropenic enterocolitis or so-called typhlitis (inflammation limited to the cecum) affects up to 10% of children under chemotherapy and presents with fever, periumbilical or generalized abdominal pain, and possible ileus. It is defined as abdominal pain with an absolute neutrophil count (ANC) of less than 500 neutrophils/ml, a core body temperature above 38.3 °C, as well as bowel wall thickening of over 4 mm in over 3 cm bowel length on imaging studies [1]. In a quarter of patients, pain is localized to the right lower quadrant, accompanied by vomiting, diarrhea, nausea, abdominal distension, and a palpable bowel mass [3]. Accompanying bloodstream infections, sepsis and bowel obstruction are frequent complications. Mortality is high and estimated between 20 and 50% [1]. Early diagnosis and the prompt initiation of broad-spectrum antibiotic therapy are crucial. Nonoperative therapy is generally successful in over 90% of cases. Initial bowel rest with restricted oral intake, fluid and electrolyte substitution, neutrophil stimulation, and close monitoring is often required as well. Should no improvement occur after 72–96 h, empiric antimycotic therapy should be considered [2]. Surgery is challenging because of impaired healing, localized and generalized inflammation, as well as vulnerable tissues. Surgical intervention should only be considered after failure of medical treatment and in cases of intestinal perforation, intra-abdominal abscesses, abdominal compartment syndrome, and persistent bleeding, accompanied by rapid clinical deterioration [3].

Differentiation between acute appendicitis and neutropenic colitis is challenging. Diagnostic errors in up to 37% of cases have been reported [5]. Imaging studies may demonstrate abdominal wall thickening, bowel wall thickening, intramural pneumatosis, periintestinal fluid collections, pneumoperitoneum, or abscesses. Immediate broad-spectrum antibiotic treatment should be started in both scenarios after obtaining blood cultures.

22.6 Anorectal Disease

Perianal disease occurs in up to 9% of neutropenic patients and usually presents in an atypical manner because neutropenia impedes the formation of classical abscesses. Cross-sectional imaging should be considered to look for possible fistulization. Digital rectal exams should only be performed cautiously due to fragile tissues and the associated traumatization of the pediatric patient. The least invasive form of therapy should be chosen with first-line treatment consisting of open drainage of superficial abscesses, as well as systemic antibiotic treatment and drain placement of deeper abscesses. More extensive surgical interventions should be postponed until neutropenia and inflammation have resolved. It is important to note that abscess formation will increase with rising neutrophil counts [1].

22.7 Intestinal Obstruction and Intussusception

Although vomiting is not uncommon in patients undergoing chemotherapy, repeated bilious emesis should raise a cause of concern, especially in combination with abdominal discomfort or pain. The presence of these symptoms calls for a thorough workup. Oncologic patients are at high risk for developing adhesions or strictures after abdominal surgery due to inflammatory and immunological imbalance. Intestinal obstruction due to tumor compression should also be ruled out, particularly in patients with neuroblastoma, nephroblastoma, abdominal lymphoma, or ovarian tumors. Mechanical obstruction needs to be distinguished from paralytic ileus, which may be caused by opioid analgesics or vinca alkaloids. In patients with intestinal obstructive symptoms, plain film abdominal radiographs should be obtained, looking for dilated bowel loops with air-fluid levels and the absence of gas distal to the obstruction [5]. A nonoperative therapeutic approach consisting of food restriction, intestinal decompression, and rehydration is initially a reasonable approach in these patients and has a success rate around 40%. In case of failure of medical management, the least invasive surgical intervention should be favored [6].

22.8 Postoperative Intussusception

A rare but relevant reason for intestinal mechanical obstruction in oncologic patients is postoperative intussusception. According to the literature, postoperative intussusception is most frequently associated with retroperitoneal tumor resection. This type of intussusception is most often ileoileal in location. The symptoms are those of intestinal obstruction but typically occur comparatively earlier than in the case of adhesive obstruction, often in the first week after the intervention. Prompt diagnosis is essential, as early therapy significantly reduces the risk of morbidity. Ultrasound can be a useful diagnostic tool with high sensitivity and specificity, although overlying gas may obscure the findings. If the ultrasound is inconclusive in the setting of worrisome symptoms, a computed tomography or magnetic resonance scan should be obtained. The typical imaging findings are the target or pseudokidney sign. If the diagnosis has been confirmed, rapid surgical reduction of the intussusception is necessary in most cases. Fortunately, bowel resection is rarely necessary and may be required in cases that are diagnosed late. In the case of transient ileoileal intussusception, watchful waiting with close sonographic follow-up in a clinically stable patient is possible [7].

One must not forget that ileocolic or ileoileal intussusception may also be the first presentation of an underlying malignant disease. In children outside of the typical age range from 2 months to 2 years, intussusception is more likely to result from a lead point structure. Therefore, malignant masses should be ruled out in such patients. Non-Hodgkin lymphoma is notorious to present this way. The surgical approach depends on the clinical presentation. If possible, bowel resection should be avoided. One option is to only perform a biopsy with possible creation of an ostomy as needed.

22.9 Intestinal Perforation

Spontaneous intestinal perforation in the child with oncologic illness is frequently associated with non-Hodgkin lymphoma. The underlying pathomechanism is transmural bowel invasion by the tumor. Perforation may result from tumor growth and displacement, as well as bowel wall necrosis caused by chemotherapy. Thus, intestinal perforation can occur both before and during chemotherapy. Perforations with associated peritonitis due to contamination of the abdomen with intestinal content pose a high risk to the already immunocompromised patient. Immunosuppressive chemotherapy makes the body more susceptible to fatal systemic infection. Intestinal perforation may lead to sepsis, prolonged hospitalization, delayed initiation or discontinuation of chemotherapy, wound healing disorders, and multiorgan failure. Decisions on the operative strategy, the extent of any necessary bowel resection, stoma formation or primary anastomosis, treatment of associated sepsis and complications, as well as timing of resumption of chemotherapy must be made based on the individual case. Primary anastomosis is possible if healthy bowel wall edges are present after tumor resection and adequate healing of the tissue can be assumed. In the case of severely damaged tissue, the creation of an enterostomy is the safer option [4].

22.10 Esophageal Stenosis and Fistulas After Chemotherapy and Radiotherapy

Long-term survival after childhood tumors is steadily increasing. Therefore, general surgical follow-up must also include dealing with the long-term complications of previous oncological treatment. Chemotherapy, radiotherapy, and stem cell transplantation can cause esophagitis, candida infections, and graft-versus-host reactions; all of them leading to potential esophageal complications. The mucosa of the esophagus can be severely affected and promote long-term esophageal stenosis. Clinically, esophageal stenosis manifests is manifested by dysphagia with or without bolus events. Contrast esophagography and endoscopy are used to confirm the diagnosis. A recent study showed that repeated endoscopic balloon dilations have a high success rate in post-chemotherapy and radiation stenoses [8]. In this study, an average of five dilations was necessary to establish long-term patency. Antirefluxive and antifungal therapies were started as supportive measures. Fortunately, the development of fistulas was rare. In those few and complex cases in which a fistula is found, temporary esophageal diversion followed by later esophagocoloplasty or gastric interposition has been described [8].

22.11 Hemorrhagic Cystitis

Hemorrhagic cystitis is not uncommon in pediatric oncologic patients with an incidence of 5 up to 70%. In children, hemorrhagic cystitis most commonly occurs shortly after the administration of certain chemotherapeutic agents, or as a long-term consequence of stem cell transplantation. In case of the latter, early-onset bleeding is mostly due to the conditioning treatment itself. The chemotherapeutics mostly associated are cyclophosphamide, ifosfamide, and busulfan. In contrast, late-onset bleeding is more often associated with reactivation of asymptomatic viruses such as BK virus, cytomegalovirus (CMV), JC virus, and adenovirus. The risk can be lowered by prophylactic treatment during chemotherapy, consisting mainly of hyperhydration, continuous bladder irrigation, and addition of mesna. In case of failure of medical treatment and the formation of large blood clots in the bladder, cystoscopy may be employed to evacuate blood clots and apply prostaglandin E1, which has been described to have cytoprotective effects in the experimental setting by regulating mucous production. In extremely refractory cases, bilateral percutaneous nephrostomy tubes might be required, based on the theory that diverting the urine from the bladder and removing the fibrinolytic activity of urokinase will promote blood clotting in the bladder and hemostasis. Emergency cystectomy is rarely indicated and should be only considered in patients with life-threatening uncontrollable bleeding [9].

22.12 Inguinal Hernia and Hydrocele

Inguinal hernia and hydrocele are common pediatric surgical conditions and thus can also affect children undergoing oncologic treatment. Intra-abdominal ascites may promote the development of an inguinal hernia. Regarding the treatment, the current literature lacks specific treatment algorithms in oncology patients. Generally, elective repair should be planned for a time when blood cell counts have recovered to allow for adequate tissue healing. Incarcerated hernias must be dealt with immediately. If manual reduction is not possible, surgical exploration and reduction are indicated. Interestingly patients with myelodysplastic syndrome or acute melodic leukemia may have a GATA-2 deficiency, which is associated with lymphedema, including hydrocele [10]. Treatment of such a patient, particularly when immunocompromised, can be challenging. In our department, it has been our experience that in such cases, repeated percutaneous relief of the fluid in the hydroceles may be a useful temporizing measure. After recovery of the blood cell counts, surgical hydrocele resection should be performed.

22.13 Priapism

Priapism is defined as the state of prolonged erection lasting longer than 4 h without any sexual stimulation. It is categorized as either low-flow or high-flow priapism. Pediatric oncologic patients present with low-flow priapism, also referred to as ischemic priapism. Childhood leukemia often causes hyperleukocytosis and thrombocytosis, leading to leukostatis in the corpus cavernosum and obstruction of the venous return. In adulthood, priapism is considered an absolute emergency. This is not the case in children, where nonoperative measures may be successful in solving the problem. Also, children seem to tolerate longer episodes of priapism better. Medical treatment consists of rehydration, addressing the underlying oncologic disease, and anticoagulation, if necessary. Additional supportive measures such as analgesia and local cooling may be useful. The next but more invasive step would be aspiration of the corpora cavernosa with or without irrigation. In our experience this was never necessary, and one should always keep in mind the risk of an invasive procedure for patients with neutropenia and immunodeficiency.

Surgeon's Checklist

1. Oncologic patients can suffer from any general pediatric emergency.
2. Illnesses might not have classical presentation.
3. Discuss treatment timing and options with the treating oncologist.
4. Transfer the patient to a center with on-site oncologists and a pediatric surgery department experienced in the treatment of oncologic patients.
5. If possible, postpone surgery until risk factors improve.
6. If there is a less invasive alternative, do not delay oncologic therapy because of surgical treatment.
7. Neutropenia is the highest risk factor for morbidity and mortality. It impedes wound healing and multiplies the risk for infection.
8. Check preoperative laboratory findings and aim to improve them before surgery.

References

1. White MG, Morgan RB, Drazer MW, Eng OS. Gastrointestinal surgical emergencies in the neutropenic immunocompromised patient. J Gastrointest Surg. 2021;25:3258–64. https://doi.org/10.1007/s11605-021-05116-9. Epub 2021 Sep 10. PMID: 34506017; PMCID: PMC8665083
2. Spiegl HR, Estepp JH, Li C, Gil S, Gosain A, Murphy AJ, Davidoff AM. Risk for deep venous thrombosis in pediatric cancer patients undergoing surgery. J Pediatr Surg. 2021;56:2360–3. https://doi.org/10.1016/j.jpedsurg.2021.01.047. Epub 2021 Feb 13
3. Cross SJ, Patel JR, Wolf J. Diagnosis and management of typhlitis and neutropenic enterocolitis in children with cancer. Pediatr Infect Dis J. 2022;41:e326–8. https://doi.org/10.1097/INF.0000000000003556. Epub 2022 Jul 13
4. Many BT, Lautz TB, Dobrozsi S, et al. Appendectomy versus observation for appendicitis in neutropenic children with cancer. Pediatrics. 2021;147(2):e2020027797. https://doi.org/10.1542/peds.2020-027797.
5. Handa A, Nozaki T, Makidono A, Okabe T, Morita Y, Fujita K, Matsusako M, Kono T, Kurihara Y, Hasegawa D, Kumamoto T, Ogawa C, Yuza Y, Manabe A. Pediatric oncologic emergencies: clinical and imaging review for pediatricians. Pediatr Int. 2019;61:122–39. https://doi.org/10.1111/ped.13755. Epub 2019 Feb 7
6. Habti M, Miyata S, Côté J, Krauel L, Piché N. Bowel obstruction following pediatric abdominal cancer surgery. Pediatr Surg Int. 2022;38:1041–5. https://doi.org/10.1007/s00383-022-05127-w. Epub 2022 Apr 16
7. VanHouwelingen LT, Seims AD, Ortega-Laureano L, Coleman JL, McCarville MB, Davidoff AM, Fernandez-Pineda I. Use of ultrasound in diagnosing postoperative small-bowel intussusception in pediatric surgical oncology patients: a single-center retrospective review. Pediatr Radiol. 2018;48:204–9. https://doi.org/10.1007/s00247-017-4018-3. Epub 2017 Oct 30
8. Lal DR, Foroutan HR, Su WT, Wolden SL, Boulad F, La Quaglia MP. The management of treatment-related esophageal complications in children and adolescents with cancer. J Pediatr Surg. 2006;41:495–9. https://doi.org/10.1016/j.jpedsurg.2005.11.065.
9. Hannick JH, Koyle MA. Canadian urological association best practice report: pediatric hemorrhagic cystitis. Can Urol Assoc J. 2019;13:E325–34. https://doi.org/10.5489/cuaj.5993. PMID: 31763977; PMCID: PMC6877374
10. Wlodarski MW, Collin M, Horwitz MS. GATA2 deficiency and related myeloid neoplasms. Semin Hematol. 2017;54:81–6. https://doi.org/10.1053/j.seminhematol.2017.05.002. Epub 2017 May 10. PMID: 28637621; PMCID: PMC5650112

23 Surgical Management of Pulmonary Metastases in Pediatric Solid Tumors

Andrew M. Davidoff

23.1 Introduction

Metastasis is the process by which cancer cells spread from a primary tumor to distant sites. It is the hallmark of malignant neoplasms and has significant therapeutic and prognostic implications. Metastatic disease is the major cause of treatment failure in cancer patients and the principal contributing factor to cancer-associated morbidity. Patients with metastatic disease may succumb to organ failure due to anatomic compromise or complications associated with the generally more intensive therapy required to treat disseminated disease. Ten to thirty percent of children with solid tumors present with metastases and an additional 15–20% relapse at distant sites [1]. Although significant progress has been made in the treatment of pediatric solid tumors, advances in the treatment of metastatic solid tumors have not mirrored those for localized disease [1]. As a disseminated process, the successful treatment of metastatic disease requires effective systemic therapy; therefore, a curative role for surgery is not intuitive, although occasionally a surgical intervention can be therapeutic. In general, the less sensitive the tumor histologic type is to adjuvant therapy, the more likely it is that metastasectomy may be beneficial. Although metastasis can occur at a variety of sites, including the lymph nodes, liver, bone, and brain, a majority of pediatric solid tumor metastases occur in the lung, and the tumors which have been shown to benefit from metastasectomy have a higher propensity to metastasize to the lung. The incidence, prognosis, and treatment for metastatic disease are histology-dependent.

The differential diagnosis for pediatric pulmonary lesions is mainly comprised of benign disease entities. However, in a patient with a history of a solid tumor, the likelihood that a new lung lesion is a metastasis is significant. Benign etiologies include infectious, congenital, atelectasis, and neoplastic. Primary lung malignancies are rare, at less than 1%. Table 23.1 shows the incidence, common site(s) of metastatic disease, and outcome for patients with newly diagnosis solid tumors.

Computed tomography (CT) scan became the gold standard for the identification of pulmonary nodules in 1979 when a prospective study by Chang et al. demonstrated the higher sensitivity of this imaging modality over plain chest radiographs [2]. CT has become even more sensitive over time with improvements in technology, and CT is still the preferred method of surveillance and identification of pulmonary nodules in children. However, the limitations of CT are still apparent in multiple pediatric solid tumors, including the fact that there are generally no findings pathognomonic for specific histologies, both

A. M. Davidoff (✉)
Department of Surgery, St. Jude Children's Research Hospital, Memphis, TN, USA
e-mail: Andrew.Davidoff@StJude.org

L. Krauel (ed.), *Survival Handbook in Pediatric Surgical Oncology*,
https://doi.org/10.1007/978-3-031-65890-7_23

Table 23.1 Metastases in pediatric solid tumors

Tumor type	Metastases at diagnosis	Sites	Survival
Neuroblastoma	60%	Bone marrow, cortical bone, lymph nodes, liver	<30%
Wilms tumor	15%	Lungs, liver	80% (FH) 17%(UH)
Rhabdomyosarcoma	10–20%	Lungs, lymph nodes, marrow	>20%
Osteosarcoma	10–20%	Lungs, bone, liver	22%
Ewing sarcoma	20–25%	Lungs, bone	<30%
Synovial sarcoma	16% synchronous	Lungs, bone	<10%
Hepatoblastoma	24% (17% to lung)	Lungs, lymph nodes, bone	40%

neoplastic and nonneoplastic, and agreement between independent reviewers is poor [3].

23.2 Surgical Approaches

There are a variety of techniques used for performing procedures on pulmonary metastases. An image-guided core needle biopsy can be performed, generally by an interventional radiologist, and is the least invasive approach. Not all lesions are amenable to this approach, however, particularly small lesions. In addition, sampling error can occur, and this approach does not offer therapeutic lesion resection. Thoracoscopic procedures are being used increasingly, as a minimally invasive method for obtaining diagnostic tissue, and, in certain circumstances, for therapeutic resection. Difficulties may arise, however, when trying to localize the CT-identified lesions. While superficial lesions can be seen intraoperatively on visual inspection and larger, firmer lesions can be palpated with instruments, many deeper, smaller, softer lesions can easily be missed. Multiple techniques have been used to overcome this problem, including preoperative marking with wires, coils, or dye and localization with intraoperative ultrasound [4]. Recently, fluorescence-guided surgery has become an increasingly used modality, particularly when localizing liver tumor metastases [5].

An open approach provides the opportunity to use tactile sensation to aid with lesion localization. Access to the chest can be achieved via a number of incisions including a posterolateral thoracotomy, with or without a muscle sparing approach, an incision in the midaxillary line, or via a sternotomy, either a median sternotomy or transverse sternotomy (clamshell). Wedge resection of individual lesions is preferred to lobectomy, when possible, to maintain maximal pulmonary reserve.

23.3 The Role of Surgery in the Management of Lung Metastases

As a disseminated process, successful treatment of metastatic disease requires effective systemic therapy. The curative role for surgery is not intuitive although occasionally it can be therapeutic. There are two general scenarios. The first is when the tumor is of a histology that is sensitive to adjuvant therapy (chemotherapy and/or radiation therapy), there is probably only a limited therapeutic role for metastasectomy, although there may be a diagnostic role. However, for tumors that are not sensitive to adjuvant therapy, there may be a therapeutic role for metastasectomy. Overall, the role of surgery in the management of patients with metastatic disease must be considered, generally, on a histology-by-histology basis (Table 23.2).

Table 23.2 Chemotherapy sensitivity of common pediatric solid tumors

Chemosensitive	Chemoresistant
Neuroblastoma	Adrenocortical carcinoma
Rhabdomyosarcoma	Non-rhabdomyosarcoma soft tissue sarcomas
Ewing sarcoma family of tumors	DSRCT (Desmoplastic Small Round Cell Tumor)
Wilms tumor	Renal cell carcinoma, rhabdoid tumor of the kidney, clear cell sarcoma
Hepatoblastoma	Hepatocellular carcinoma
Germ cell tumors	Malignant thymoma

23.4 Osteosarcoma

Osteosarcoma is the most common pediatric bone tumor, with 400 new cases per year in the USA. Twenty percent of these patients present with metastasis at diagnosis, and another 20% eventually develop metastasis. Pulmonary metastases comprise 85% of these metastases. Numerous studies have shown that complete surgical resection of primary and metastatic disease is essential for cure.

Given the premise that surgical tumor clearance is needed for cure, the surgical approach to pulmonary metastasectomy in osteosarcoma is a source of much debate. The use of an open technique with exploration and palpation of both lungs has been supported by evidence that complete resection of all detectable disease is necessary for survival, preoperative CT misses up to a quarter of viable osteosarcoma metastases found by palpation [6], and by evidence that up to 60% of patients with unilateral CT lesions have contralateral metastases at exploration [7]. However, it has never been proven that removal of lesions not seen on CT changes patient outcome. A current randomized Children's Oncology Group (COG) trial is underway to look at outcomes of thoracoscopy versus thoracotomy. A retrospective study by Fernandez Pineda et al. has already suggested that in selected cases where only one nodule is seen on CT scan, a minimally invasive approach to nodule removal will be sufficient, as these patients are likely to have only the one pathologic lung nodule [8].

Several options exist for clearing disease in both lungs. One can perform a sternotomy, either a median sternotomy or a transverse sternotomy. This has the benefit of being a single operation to access both lungs, and it may be associated with less postoperative pain. It has the potential disadvantage that lung lesions that are posterior, multiple, and large in the left lower lobe may be hard to approach. Another alternative is bilateral sequential thoracotomies, performed during a single anesthetic. This provides good exposure but requires a longer operative and anesthetic time. Lastly, staged bilateral thoracotomies can be performed. This provides optimal exposure of each hemithorax and avoids a longer operative and anesthetic time but does have the disadvantage of delay in removing all disease. Although survival is increasingly worse with each successive recurrence, there still is some benefit to performing multiple thoracotomies for lung-only relapses in terms of survival, if complete resection is possible. Survivors of single or multiple thoracotomies for metastasectomy generally experience only mild long-term decrease in pulmonary function [9].

23.5 Non-rhabdomyosarcoma Soft Tissue Sarcoma

The lungs are the most common site for metastasis of non-rhabdomyosarcoma soft tissue sarcomas (NRSTS). Subtypes that most commonly metastasize to the lung include synovial sarcoma, alveolar soft part sarcoma, chondrosarcoma, high-grade fibrosarcoma, and malignant fibrous histiocytoma. Metastases from NRSTS generally do not respond well to whole-lung irradiation or chemotherapy; therefore, the surgical approach is similar to that of osteosarcoma. However, intraoperative lesion identification and localization are often more difficult because, unlike osteosarcoma where there is osteoid matrix, metastatic NRSTS lung lesions tend to be softer and may feel like a collapsed lung. There are data to suggest that pulmonary metastasectomy is associated with improved survival in patients with metastatic synovial sarcoma and alveolar soft part sarcoma, in particular, if complete resection is achieved.

23.6 Rhabdomyosarcoma/Ewing Sarcoma

Rhabdomyosarcoma and Ewing sarcoma, where 20% of patients present with metastatic disease, most commonly in the lung, are both considered to be histologies that are sensitive to adjuvant therapy; therefore, surgical resection is generally not recommended as it does not clearly improve the poor survival for these patients. Surgery is generally limited to biopsy for diagnostic purposes or removal of isolated stable lesions, although the role of surgery for each continues to be assessed in the Children's Oncology Group (COG).

23.7 Wilms Tumor

Ten percent of children with Wilms tumor have lung metastases at diagnosis. Despite the presence of metastatic disease, if the histology is favorable, there is an 80% survival for these patients because favorable histology Wilms tumor is sensitive to adjuvant therapy, generally consisting of three drug chemotherapy (vincristine, actinomycin D, and doxorubicin) and radiation. Because of this, there historically has been little role for surgery in the management of metastatic, favorable histology Wilms tumor. However, there may now be an expanding role for surgery, at least in the form of diagnostic biopsy. Biopsy of lung lesions of uncertain significance seen on initial chest CT may assist in determining whether a patient has metastatic disease. Additionally, a recent clinical trial performed by the Children's Oncology Group demonstrated the usefulness of an algorithm whereby patients with lung metastases whose lung disease disappeared by imaging after 6 weeks of three drug chemotherapy were declared "rapid responders" and radiation therapy was no longer recommended. Those with an incomplete response by imaging at week 6 were considered "slow incomplete responders" and not only went on to have adjuvant lung radiation but also had chemotherapy intensified [10]. Surgery may be performed to determine whether or not residual nodules seen on imaging contained viable Wilms tumor and, potentially, reclassify patients as rapid responders. However, currently, surgical clearance of residual, viable disease in the lung does not obviate the need for lung irradiation. There is only a 17% survival in patients with metastatic anaplastic Wilms tumor as this histologic subtype is generally refractory to adjuvant therapy. Because of this, there may be a role for surgery to render these patients clinically disease-free prior to stem cell transplant.

23.8 Liver Tumors

The most common liver tumors in children are hepatoblastoma and hepatocellular carcinoma (HCC). Both metastasize to the lung in about 20% of cases at diagnosis. These two histologies are very different in their sensitivity to adjuvant therapy, and, therefore, the role of pulmonary metastasectomy is different. Hepatoblastoma is very sensitive to adjuvant therapy, whereas HCC is not. So, for hepatoblastoma, resection of metastatic disease is rarely indicated although disease isolated to the lung, persisting after adjuvant therapy, may benefit from resection and is associated with an improved event-free survival [11]. Resection of residual lung disease may also allow these patients to be eligible for liver transplant in situations where this is required for local control. Serum alpha fetoprotein is an excellent tumor marker that is helpful in detecting and determining the nature of residual or recurrent pulmonary nodules and for follow-up. HCC, because of its adjuvant therapy refractory nature, may benefit from resection of lung metastases in selected patients, as it may prolong survival.

23.9 Neuroblastoma

Over 60% of patients with neuroblastoma have metastases at presentation, but rarely do they have pulmonary metastases at that time. Lung metastases generally occur only in patients with end-stage disease, and so pulmonary metastasectomy is rarely indicated.

23.10 Germ Cell Tumors

Germ cell tumors are known to be very sensitive to three-drug chemotherapy which includes cisplatin, etoposide, and bleomycin, with excellent long-term survival. The lung is the most frequent site of distant metastases in these patients, but metastasectomy is rarely indicated. Residual lesions seen on imaging studies performed after completion of adjuvant therapy may harbor viable tumor although the majority will be either fibrosis, necrosis, or mature teratoma. The role of pulmonary metastasectomy in these circumstances is to determine if there is viable tumor in lesions after chemotherapy and, thus, if additional or different therapy is needed.

23.11 Adrenocortical Carcinoma

Adrenocortical carcinoma (ACC) is a rare disease in children but has a 7% incidence of pulmonary metastases at presentation. Complete surgical excision is critical as effective adjuvant therapies are not available. Pulmonary metastasectomy may improve survival, at least based on adult literature, although, overall survival for children with metastatic ACC is very poor.

23.12 Thyroid Cancer

Thyroid cancer is another rare pediatric malignancy although it makes up 8% of second malignant neoplasms. There is a 20% incidence of distant metastases primarily to the lung in patients with thyroid cancer. Thyroid cancer in children has an indolent course with excellent survival of over 95% and is even over 85% in patients with metastatic disease. Therapeutic radioactive iodine is effective for metastatic disease; therefore, pulmonary metastasectomy is only done if the histology of a pulmonary lesion is uncertain, especially after I131 radiotherapy.

23.13 Conclusions

Almost 30 percent of children and adolescents with solid tumors will present with metastatic disease, most often in the lung. Others with initially localized disease will relapse in the lung. General principles when considering pulmonary metastasectomy include having local control and removal of all disease if the histology is one which is insensitive to adjuvant therapies. The role of surgery is clearly histology-dependent. A central role has been confirmed only for osteosarcoma although there is likely a survival benefit for patients with non-rhabdomyosarcoma soft tissue sarcomas. For other histologies, surgery generally has only a diagnostic role although solitary persistent nodules may benefit especially if there is no effective adjuvant therapy.

Surgeon Checklist

Before embarking on a pulmonary metastasectomy, consider:

1. Has local control been established?
2. Is the purpose diagnostic or therapeutic?
3. Is the tumor histology chemosensitive, radiosensitive, both, or neither?
4. Are the metastases limited to the lung or widespread throughout other tissues?
5. Would preoperative localizing techniques be helpful in identifying the lesion(s)?
6. Do both chests need to be explored and is this best done with one operation or two?

During the operation, consider:

7. What is the optimal surgical approach (e.g., open vs. minimally invasive)?
8. What is the optimal incision for approaching all lesions?
9. How can the lesion(s) be removed to spare the greatest amount of normal parenchyma?
10. Is there any role for frozen section analysis before removing all lesions?

References

1. Fuchs J, Seitz G, Handgretinger R, Schäfer J, Warmann SW. Surgical treatment of lung metastases in patients with embryonal pediatric solid tumors: an update. Semin Pediatr Surg. 2012;21(1):79–87.
2. Chang AE, Schaner EG, Conkle DM, Flye MW, Doppman JL, Rosenberg SA. Evaluation of computed tomography in the detection of pulmonary metastases: a prospective study. Cancer. 1979;43(3):913–6.
3. McCarville MB, Lederman HM, Santana VM, Daw NC, Shochat SJ, Li CS, et al. Distinguishing benign from malignant pulmonary nodules with helical chest CT in children with malignant solid tumors. Radiology. 2006;239(2):514–20.
4. Morgan K, Anderson K, Crowley J, Johnston M. Interhospital variability in localization techniques for small pulmonary nodules in children: a pediatric surgical oncology research collaborative study. J Pediatr Surg. 2022;57:1013–7.
5. Abdelhafeez AH, Mothi SS, Pio L, Mori M, Santiago TC, McCarville MB, et al. Feasibility of indocyanine green-guided localization of pulmonary nodules in children with solid tumors. Pediatr Blood Cancer. 2023;70:e30437.
6. Heaton TE, Hammond WJ, Farber BA, Pallos V, Meyers PA, Chou AJ, et al. A 20-year retrospective analysis of CT-based pre-operative identification of pulmonary metastases in patients with osteosarcoma: a single-center review. J Pediatr Surg. 2017;52(1):115–9.
7. Su WT, Chewning J, Abramson S, Rosen N, Gholizadeh M, Healey J, et al. Surgical management and outcome of osteosarcoma patients with unilateral pulmonary metastases. J Pediatr Surg. 2004;39(3):418–23. discussion 418–23
8. Fernandez-Pineda I, Daw NC, McCarville B, Emanus LJ, Rao BN, Davidoff AM, et al. Patients with osteosarcoma with a single pulmonary nodule on computed tomography: a single-institution experience. J Pediatr Surg. 2012;47(6):1250–4.
9. Denbo JW, Zhu L, Srivastava D, Stokes DC, Srinivasan S, Hudson MM, et al. Long-term pulmonary function after metastasectomy for childhood osteosarcoma: a report from the St Jude lifetime cohort study. J Am Coll Surg. 2014;219(2):265–71.
10. Dix DB, Seibel NL, Chi YY, Khanna G, Gratias E, Anderson JR, et al. Treatment of stage IV favorable histology Wilms tumor with lung metastases: a report from the Children's oncology group AREN0533 study. J Clin Oncol. 2018;36(16):1564–70.
11. Fleming AM, Murphy AJ, Sarvode Mothi S, Interiano RB, Loh A, McCarville ME, et al. Aggressive pursuit of no evidence of disease status in hepatoblastoma improves survival: an observational study. J Pediatr Surg. 2023;58(6):1081–7.

The Role of the Surgeon in Palliative Care

24

Israel Fernandez-Pineda

24.1 Introduction

Palliative surgery is often defined as a surgical intervention with intent to improve a patient's quality of life by relieving suffering secondary to symptoms of advanced disease. It remains the obligation of the pediatric surgeon to act in the best interest of the patient and to determine, in conjunction with the patient, the family, and other caregivers, what the best interests might be. Handling such conflicts can be difficult because pediatric surgeons may have limited training in palliative care. There is limited literature that specifically addresses the role of the pediatric surgeon in palliative care [1]. Surgeons are sometimes consulted later in the course of disease with the hope that they can provide a life-saving or life-prolonging procedure on a terminally ill child. The surgeon is considered to be the last hope to regain, if not cure, some sense of normalcy for a period of time. Ethics consultation should be considered to facilitate discussion of these complex issues. Providers cannot be forced to deliver care that they do not think is indicated or beneficial [2]. It is critical to review the goals of the patient and family and to determine which goals are attainable. The goals of care must be clearly defined when considering surgical interventions. There are times when procedures are not appropriate. These conversations can be difficult for the surgeon and unbearable for parents who want to believe that they are doing everything possible for their child. Pediatric surgery trainees experience ethical distress in the rendering of care for critically ill patients, especially with regard to end-of-life issues. Few surgical training programs have formal mentorship arrangements for trainees, yet this may provide trainees with an effective means to voice personal concerns, to seek clinical advice, and to address unresolved moral conflicts.

During the decision-making process, there are less and more challenging situations (Fig. 24.1). Less challenging decision-making situations include those circumstances when the patient/family insists on a surgical procedure that is neither safe nor indicated. The surgeon should explain to the patient/family why this procedure is not indicated and the potential negative consequences. Also, when the patient/family refuses a surgical procedure, a surgeon must respect that decision. More challenging decision-making situations are more common as they represent a large gray scale of clinical scenarios where multiple factors play an important role.

I. Fernandez-Pineda (✉)
Department of Paediatric Surgery, Children's Health Ireland at Crumlin, Dublin, Ireland

L. Krauel (ed.), *Survival Handbook in Pediatric Surgical Oncology*,
https://doi.org/10.1007/978-3-031-65890-7_24

If a patient/family with decision-making capacity insists on a **surgery that is neither safe nor idicated,** a surgeon must refuse to provide the requested treatment	GRAY SCALE	If a patient/family with decision-making capacity insists on a **refuses surgery,** a surgeon must respect the patient´s autonomy and cannot forcé a treatment on that patient
Less challenging decision making	More challenging decision making	Less challenging decision making

Fig. 24.1 Challenges in decision-making

24.2 Surgical Procedures for Palliative Care

Surgical procedures are sometimes necessary to control symptoms such as pain, dyspnea from fluid collection, urinary/intestinal obstruction, hemorrhage, and cachexia. Some examples of these procedures include:

(a) Image-guided nerve block and amputation.
(b) Thoracostomy and pleurodesis.
(c) Gastrostomy.
(d) Tracheostomy.

24.2.1 Image-Guided Nerve Blockade and Amputation

Nerve block can provide pain relief with minimally invasive techniques guided by ultrasound or computed tomography (CT) imaging. Procedures can be repeated as needed by the patient. This is particularly helpful in intractable extremity sarcomas that invade nerve roots or peripheral nerves. Celiac plexus neurolysis may be helpful for pain relief in patients with abdominal pain from unresectable abdominal tumors.

Palliative amputation in children with a limited life expectancy by improving pain, mobility, and psychological and emotional well-being may play a role in the management of end-of-life events. Merimsky et al. found that severely ill or debilitated patients with metastatic musculoskeletal disease were likely to opt for major limb amputation [3]. In these patients who had low chances of survival, amputations improved the ability to carry on daily activities; significantly alleviated pain, improved emotional, sexual, and social lives; and increased the overall quality of life. Gil et al. concluded that limb amputation in children with metastatic sarcoma and limited life expectancy may be beneficial to alleviate symptoms of local disease and improve mobility, pain, and psychological and emotional well-being [4]. These findings are critical to improve patient outcomes by helping clinicians more readily discuss the role of amputation in this patient population.

24.2.2 Gastrostomy

Palliative gastrostomy tube placement is performed to establish enteral access for the administration of medications or nutrition or for venting to relieve or provide comfort from an intestinal blockage. Tube feedings through a gastrostomy or other temporary feeding tube provide comfort, but patients and parents should understand that providing enteral feeds cannot reverse the metabolic process of cachexia. Lack of nutrition may be beneficial at the end of life because it promotes ketosis and endorphin production; decreases nausea, emesis, diarrhea, and coughing; and increases respiratory secretions and urine output.

24.2.3 Thoracostomy and Pleurodesis

Malignant pleural effusion from pediatric malignancies is an unusual problem in pediatric palliative care. Potential procedures to alleviate symptoms include repeated needle aspirations, pleurodesis with doxycycline, and insertion of chest tubes. In weighing the risks and benefits of intervention, patients and parents must be advised that the chest tubes produce pain and pleurodesis is not always successful in preventing reaccumulation of malignant effusions. Hoffer et al. found decreased respiratory rates and improved aeration following ultrasound (US)-guided pleurodesis using doxycycline as a sclerosing agent in children with cancer [5]. Portable devices may be preferable to promote patient independence and home care. In some instances, tunneled pleural catheters may be offered as they are advantageous as long-term drainage solutions.

24.2.4 Tracheostomy

This procedure is typically performed for patients who have difficulty in swallowing or maintaining their airway, or who experience recurrent aspiration events. For patients with deconditioning or other physiologic decline, tracheostomy may permit the patient to maintain or resume a certain quality of life. Tracheostomy may also permit caregivers to safely transition care for the patient to an outpatient setting. Potential complications include air leak at the surgical site and infection.

24.3 Role of Interventional Radiology

Some patients may require interventional strategies for pain control, including neuroaxial or peripheral nerve blocks, neurolysis, and ablation of painful lesions. Anghelescu et al. reported decreased pain and opioid requirements at the end of life using continuous catheter-delivered analgesia without complications for long periods of time [4]. CT-guided tumor ablation, with either radiofrequency or cryoablation, has shown therapeutic outcomes to relieve pain from tumor in children with benign and malignant lesions with several advantages such as more rapid pain reduction, shorter hospital stay, and more prolonged analgesic effect.

Surgeon's Checklist

1. The surgeon, as a part of the interdisciplinary collaboration, should act in the best interest of the patient and to determine, in conjunction with the patient, the family, and other caregivers, what the best interests might be.
2. Less invasive image-guided procedures usually performed by interventional radiologists are occasionally preferred to invasive surgical procedures.
3. There is limited literature that specifically addresses the role of the pediatric surgeon in palliative care.
4. The surgeon is considered to be the last hope to regain, if not cure, some sense of normalcy for a period of time.
5. Ethics consultation should be considered to facilitate discussion of these complex issues.
6. Nerve block can provide pain relief with minimally invasive techniques guided by ultrasound or CT imaging.
7. Palliative amputation in children with a limited life expectancy by improving pain, mobility, and psychological and emotional well-being may play a role in the management of end-of-life events.

References

1. Inserra A, Narciso A, Paolantonio G, Messina R, Crocoli A. Palliative care and pediatric surgical oncology. Semin Pediatr Surg. 2016;25(5):323–32.
2. Moroney MR, Lefkowits C. Evidence for integration of palliative care into surgical oncology practice and education. J Surg Oncol. 2019;120(1):17–22.
3. Merimsky O, Kollender Y, Inbar M, et al. Palliative treatment for advanced or metastatic osteosarcoma. Isr Med Assoc J. 2004;6(1):34–8.
4. Gil S, Fernandez-Pineda I, Rao B, Neel MD, Baker JN, Wu H, Wu J, Anghelescu DL. Role of amputation in improving mobility, pain outcomes, and emotional and psychological Well-being in children with metastatic osteosarcoma. Am J Hosp Palliat Care. 2019;36(2):105–10.
5. Hoffer FA, Hancock ML, Hinds PS, Oigbokie N, Rai SN, Rao B. Pleurodesis for effusions in pediatric oncology patients at end of life. Pediatr Radiol. 2007;37(3):269–73.

MIX
Papier aus verantwortungsvollen Quellen
Paper from responsible sources
FSC® C105338

If you have any concerns about our products,
you can contact us on
ProductSafety@springernature.com

In case Publisher is established outside the EU,
the EU authorized representative is:
Springer Nature Customer Service Center GmbH
Europaplatz 3, 69115 Heidelberg, Germany

Printed by Libri Plureos GmbH
in Hamburg, Germany